DRIPFEED

By Lami Okrekson

The mental health publisher
Empowering and informing

Lami Okrekson

All rights reserved, no part of this publication may be reproduced by any means, electronic, mechanical photocopying, documentary, film or in any other format without prior written permission of the publisher.

> Published by
> Chipmunkapublishing
> PO Box 6872
> Brentwood
> Essex CM13 1ZT
> United Kingdom

http://www.chipmunkapublishing.com

Copyright © Lami Okrekson 2008

Edited by Mary Dow and Kimberley Bishop

DRIPFEED

Don't you care for my love? She said bitterly.

I handed her the mirror, and said:
Please address these questions to the proper person!
Please make all requests to the headquarters!
In all matters of emotional importance
please approach the supreme authority direct!
So I handed her the mirror

And she would have broken it over my head,
but she caught sight of her own reflection
and that held her spellbound for two seconds
while I fled.

Intimates D.H. Lawrence

Lami Okrekson

DRIPFEED

Prologue

They never taught us about contraception in school, so while half of us are up to our elbows in baby shit, the other half still fuck standing up – whatever that's supposed to do. Also, they failed miserably at our preparation for 'something else.' So the people who managed to escape the babies and the sex ended up as social retards. The ones you never see because you're not looking close enough. People who wear brown and blend into the background. You'd trip over them if they weren't so alert.

Then there's the inbetweeners, like me, who drift along not really fitting in anywhere. We are Chippers. Fifteen year olds who drink Jack Daniels for breakfast, eighteen year olds already bypassing the dragon and going straight for the veins. Primary school taught us not to fear needles. We are a nation of insomniacs and we walk around with our stoned eyes closed, or bulging out of heads that are filled with so much crap there isn't anymore room in there for education. Education sucks, we are too cool for school.

We decided we were too cool for school today and came here instead. I walk along Waterloo Bridge with Ezra. The freezing bridge where all the cold wind from the Thames blows into our chapped faces. This shit doesn't affect me as it should, considering we have been so desensitized by

Britain's weather by now. More than just a little bit of sun in summer would shock me more than this. A couple of seagulls fly overhead, shrieking their obscenities into the air. The seagulls annoy me; I don't understand why they're here, in the middle of London when they're supposed to be coasting the borders of Brighton or Margate. Seagulls in London? This is more than my head can handle. They glide along the top of the dirty, choppy water, so dirty yet so enticing - and I wish I could jump in there and float around with the carcasses of the dead fish for a while. In any case the salt water would maybe relieve this fucking constipation; I've had it for weeks, rock hard pellets of shit that refuse to dislodge themselves from my arse long enough for me to take a satisfying shit.

"We should go there one day," Ezra points towards the Hayward Gallery across from us, disrupting my thoughts, distracting me from the ache in my bowels. I nod. We will never go there though, it isn't on our cards.

We walk slowly because we have nowhere to go; also we are flying higher than British Airways. We don't show it though, our pinned pupils, that would be way too obvious.

"It's bare cold," Ezra says.

"Yeah it's cold." So what? We should know that by now.

As we walk we intercept random looks from random people also walking the bridge. They are looking at us because we are inbetweeners. They must also be inbetweeners. We can recognise

DRIPFEED

each other a mile off through a blanket of London sky. These random inbetweeners are people we've seen before, pieces of the people we hate. With their pristine suits and shinier than shiny shoes; men who look more like a Gillette commercial than real life, or women with huge ankles and tiny waists. Proportion is a phenomenon lost on the twenty first century. These are the people tourists come to London to take pictures of. There are a few of them here now, taking pictures of the river Thames. And I feel like shouting 'what the fuck!! Why are you taking pictures of a dirty river?? Don't you know where you are?' I'd never say this though. I wouldn't want to be the bad impression that put London at the bottom of 'tourist hotspots' with Arizona and Wyoming.

We watch the people on the bridge. People watching. People watching people watching people watching us. They stare at our cigarettes and our faces, thinking we are way too young for that shit. Not realising that we're travelling backwards all the time. We're always getting younger, every year. We have lost the ability to grow.
 The people we like best are the disproportionate women though, the ones with the huge ankles and tiny waists. They don't seem to care that their ankles are too fat, or that people are laughing at the fact that their feet just will not fit into their shoes. Mostly though, we like the other women, the ones who have it the other way

around; fat women with tiny ankles. These women look as though they're about to crumble and crack, as if ankles that small could never support a body that fat. It is impossible and it makes me think these women aren't filled with fat, but with air. Their tiny ankles are really the leaden weights keeping them reigned in to this life. Without them they'd just float away – like Judy Garland – over that proverbial rainbow.

These are the women I like best. They seem like some kind of neo-existentialist. Women like that couldn't possibly have husbands at home, waiting for dinner on the table, or screaming kids under their skirts. Women like that seem, to me, free. Fuck beauty; I want to be just like that when my ankles become too skinny to support my obesity.

Later, Ezra and I go back to my house. My parents are out. Or at least Stella is – out cold that is. My father is always out.

Ezra and I lay on my bed. He pulls out a bag of coke and we do a couple of lines off an old Michael Jackson record – it's so dusty it's a miracle it still plays. Belle and Chris are always saying I shouldn't do coke. I agree. I don't coke like normal people, I coke and lay passively on my bed, revelling in the slow buzz and calm muteness of the world it brings. Like the sound the world makes as it spins on its axis. Gentle and numbingly relaxing.

I was normal before Chris and Belle.

DRIPFEED

Before them I was just as fucked up as any other teenager; but I was okay. Back then it was just me and Ezra. We went to gigs, we smoked Marlboro Lights (then switched to straight Marlboros after realising 'lights' is just a word used to entice fat people), riding in cars with people we didn't know. We reminded me of the sixties; all those hippy wagons carting stoned teenagers to Jimi Hendrix.

I lay on the bed whilst Ezra takes pictures of me holding the cigarette, looking all dazed and confused. If I ever make it into suited-and-booted corporate London these will be the debilitating images that wrench me from my platform of success and land me in a gutter, or out under a bridge somewhere. The coke stings my brains as it goes up there, like pepper I'd imagine – except I've never inhaled pepper so I wouldn't really know. After the fifth line I know I've done way too much. With the windows open I should at least be able to hear the rushing of wind against tree, but the cocaine clouds me and I hear nothing.

I can't move at all and my face is so numb it feels like I've been pumped full of Novocain. From where I am laying, drooling onto the pillowcases, I have a good view of Ezra. His slim fingers deftly roll a spliff, moving swiftly between the weed and the rizla, and then the quick motions of actually sealing the thing shut. He has the hands of a guitarist; graceful but dry and peely-looking - so unlike mine, which have never graced the strings of a guitar. I don't like my hands; in fact, I don't like hands at all. Not when they're this close to my face. And there are so many hands, so many hands all in my face that I can't even see Ezra anymore. Even though he's right next to me I just can't find him, he's supposed to be on the bed next to me, except he isn't. I'm not even on the bed next to me. I'm comatose.

"Charlotte!"
"Don't fucking call me that bitch!"
"Chuck."
"What the fuck!"

This is routine. Stella and I go through it every time I OD. You'd think I had enough sense to OD once, realise I didn't actually like it that much, and promise never to do it again. Except it's all relative, to my predicament, and I am an idiot.
We were unlucky. It seems that God didn't like us too much. It's the only way I can think of to explain why Stella is such a nutso, and why daddy's been AWOL for the past sixteen years. It's the only way to explain me away; why I'm here on this bed, lacking in the energy to function for myself. Why I can't even remember if I have a sister or a brother – if I even have a sibling at all.

"You know that's bad for you." Girl! Alice.

So it's a sister I have. And I know that she infuriates me. Kids infuriate me – Period – How they always sound like they're repeating what some adult told them.

"Mum's *pissed* off at you," the sister says, in those whining intonations of the young. She

DRIPFEED

stresses the 'pissed,' like she's really proud to say it. Proud that, once again, she came out as the good one while I came out here to be examined.

"Whatever!" So fucking what. It's me, it's him, it's the world. I'm just the last excuse in a long list of excuses. It's not even insulting anymore.

Silence.

I'm lying on my own bed with a cigarette and a bottle of Jack Daniels. Ezra and Chris are doing lines on the floor. It feels like a jump-cut; like I jumped from one part of my life where it's the same but framed differently. Like, Chris and Belle weren't here before, and now they are. And I feel like the bit that happened before, in the hospital, was just an interruption in the narrative of my life. A break put in to entertain; so I could be gazed upon by a bunch of androids in white jackets.

From where I'm lying on the bed I can just see the top of Belle's peroxide head. I can't see her face properly because the Jack Daniels bottle is in the way, and her face is all liquidy and distorted. I can still tell it's her though, maybe because I know it already; like 2x2=4. There's no point in trying to understand why it is, it just is. Or like me and my life, a blank textbook of inspiration.

"You're such a loser Chuck. I mean, OD'ing again and not even giving us front row seats," Chris says to me.

"Fuck off Dildo," I say back. Chris thinks OD'ing is cool. He thinks it is what will take him from teen obscurity into socialite nirvana.

"Getting a bit rude aren't we?" He jibes.

"You think that was rude?" I say. "Then I think you'd be pretty offended if I said your hair looked like a beehive. Or that you – Belle – have a golf ball of a spot on your face. I mean you could climb that and plant a flag on top. And you," I go for Ezra. "Could you be any shorter? No, because then you'd need a stepladder to press the bell on the bus." I go for Chris again, hating him for hating me so much he has to rip me to shreds when I am so fragile. "Ugly and stupid. You must be pissed at God." I say this vehemently; insulting every one of my friends. The worst thing is they seem to think I was joking. I wasn't. I was deadly fucking serious. The world pissed me off today and I got even.

Someone like me must be so tiresome, so draining, sucking all the life out of everything. How do my friends put up with me? How do they not grow tired of the depressive blackouts and the consistent unhappy face? I'm being neutral! This is my neutral face; I can't help it if that isn't aesthetically pleasing enough for them. Shit! I'm trying my best.

But I don't understand. I honestly do not understand what people see in me, why they want to befriend me. Why they want to call me at all hours of the morning, inviting me places and taking me places. The bottom line is – the underlying question I need to ask myself everyday – why do they like me? What is special about me that they are willing to overlook all this crazy stuff?

DRIPFEED

What points can I possibly have that are so good they outweigh even my moods? Always my mood, never black, but never sunshine yellow and glowing at the edges like burning clouds. I just can't seem to find that balance. Either I'm too much or not enough. Too over-the-top, too quiet, or just not eccentric enough.

Maybe that's it; maybe this is my big problem. I'm eccentric, but not kooky enough to be considered a threat. And this brings me back, always going backwards, to why they even like me anyway. Why bother with me when there are other, more eccentric, more real, people than I am out there. I'm fake. I'm just boring and recluse.

Then it comes back to Chris. How he's here, how I annoy him so much with my overdoses and my outbursts, but he's here! He tolerates me. Why?

Chris is the only one capable of dragging me down from my mountainous pedestal. So far down, in fact, that I crash, rock bottom, on the floor at his feet. I am thoroughly dragged, shattered windows, spilt coffee, the works. I shouldn't have expected less, this is Chris all over. I shouldn't have expected more either. Without looking at him I know he is muttering some disappointment or other. Disappointed that I was the one with the attention and not him.

Gradually my friends are filtered out through the cracks in the walls, and I am left to deal with this alone. The sounds of Stella sobbing into her anti-depressants in the other room. I can feel Alice walking around this place somewhere, in a frayed sweater no doubt, leaking cuttings from Argos magazines across the floor as she goes. A sink, a bathroom, a wedding dress. Alice cuts these things out and Pritt Sticks them into blue, lined textbooks she gets from school. These are things she will need when she's older, I imagine, when she's grown-up and married. Practical. Everything about Alice is practical; from her über-thick geek glasses to her huge jumpers (they keep the warm in during the winter).

We live in a world where practicality prevails over social relevance; and Alice is about as socially relevant as a single grain of salt. Even her name is good and practical, like mine should be.

I spend a few days like this, recovering, lying atop a duvet smoking, or following behind Alice's trail of Argos and Pritt Stick remains. We stay out of direct sunlight, it hurts our eyes or we melt, I forget which. Everything hurts our eyes, the sun, the smog, the wind. It's funny, how these things always come in threes; the three Musketeers, the three wise men, the three blind mice. If the three mice were blind then we were their cataracts. Not only do we melt in sunlight, we block it out also. Three is not a magic number.

Finally, sleep wraps me in his arms and I let go of everything that had the audacity to fuck me over the last couple of years. I wake up three weeks later, and I am refreshed.

DRIPFEED

"What are you? Hmm? Because you look like my daughter, you even resemble *me* slightly, but you're not real. You're poison, like ivy. I don't know who you are; I don't even know what you are. And *you*. I've never even seen you before. Why are you here? Hmm? You must be the scum they were talking about on the news."

My mother, Stella fucking psycho-bitch, crazy as a psychologist's fucking wet dream. Having a drunken, pill-popped go at Ezra and me. It hurts me, though I never expected it would. The words stab like knives, and we are forced to move sideways to avoid them.

"So go ahead and do it," she continues.

I realise I must have blocked her out because it sounds as though I have missed some vital point of her sentence. "Get out if you want, see if I care." She grabs Alice, who just happens to be wandering close by, ready for Stella to grab and prove her point. "We don't need you, your sister and me. We can get along fine without you. We can do whatever we want if…"

Ezra and I gently back away here. Stella is drying up and, although I feel sorry for Alice, pinned to her side like that, there is nothing I want to do, except get fucked-up and dance like nobody's watching in a room full of people. We head up to my room, which is redolent of the incense I burned earlier; I was going for the whole Zen Buddhist thing, though I failed – I still like the smell though.

This time we don't do any drugs since we don't have any to do. We just lie on my bed smoking Marlboros and staring at the white foam tiles on the ceiling. Stella is still ranting to Alice about me downstairs; we can hear her through all this brick.

There is a club we always go to, Ezra and Charlie, Belle and I. Some seedy little underground dive, where skinny emo boys mosh, get beaten up by bigger emo boys – also moshing – and end up being taken away in ambulances.
    We like this club; it is good for blocking out the voices in our heads. Voices of our parents, our teachers, our psychopathic, megalomaniac inner selves. We walk to this place from Waterloo Bridge. Or rather, we cross the bridge to get to this place. It is hidden on the wrong side of the bridge, the part you look at through the window of a train, and think how lucky you are not to live there.
    We hear the music before we even see the lights; music that sounds far away, but as though it is still loud enough to penetrate the bricks and mortar between us and it. It vibrates the air around us and guides us to the door. As always, it is Ezra and I versus Charlie and Belle. Ezra and I in trench coats to hide our stashes, and shades to hide the damage.
    Charlie and Belle meet us at the door; in leather jackets to hide their coke, and ski hats to look cool. As much as I dislike them both, they are cool. We are too cool, even, for this place; with its low ceilings and dirty back rooms. We could do so much better than this.

DRIPFEED

"Nice Jacket," Belle says. Her voice drips with sarcasm. While I try to avoid all the bullshit spewing from her mouth, I look over her shoulder and notice a new girl leaning against the wall next to Charlie. He is obviously in love with her, the way he's slouching back, trying to look all hetero and masculine. We are a nation of bad posture, we slouch therefore we are.

"Where'd you get it?" she asks, her eyes never leaving mine.

"You could never afford it," I say. "So there'd be no point in telling you."

"Ah no need to get so touchy," she says. "You know I'm only fucking with you." She hugs me then, trying to disguise all this from Ezra and Charlie, and the new girl in the corner. "Come on," she continues. "I was joking, you know that."

I have never liked Belle, this girl who appears in and out of my life from time to time. The only reason I allow her at all is because she is Charlie's bitch, and Charlie is Ezra's bitch. And Ezra is mine. We are drawn to this circle purely by circumstance, it wouldn't fall apart if one of us weren't in it, but it wouldn't be the same either.

I'm not used to new people, they disturb the balance. We are a group of veterans; new people could never survive amongst us. This is why the girl disarms me momentarily. It's hard to understand why she would want to be here, where she came from, what she is going to add to us; or take away. Even though I can hardly see through all the smoke and dark, I try to gauge this new girl from where she sits opposite me. Our usual hangout, somewhere at the end of the club; two black armchairs and a leather sofa near the bar. It's funny, how no one but us ever comes here, we'd probably allow them if they did; behind our shades we are cowards.

I have only ever seen this place once during the day, and it was huge. It feels so much smaller at night, on account of all the smoke and the people and the dark. There is a hot bartender, I know, at the bar next to me, but I can't be bothered to move my head that far around; and besides, I'm still trying to suss this intruder out. She's kind of pretty, I can see why Charlie would want to make her his fag hag, but she looks crazy. It's dark, and I'm stoned, but I'm straight enough to see this crazy look in her eye. Then I start to think that maybe it's just me. This girl is sitting perfectly still, not moving not speaking; only looking. I am the crazy one in this equation; especially since there is smoke coming out of the top of Charlie's ski hat now.

"Who are you?" I say.
"Maria."
Maria, or whatever her name is, lights a cigarette that Charlie slips from his pocket and into her mouth. She blows smoke rings at me, up over our seats.

After a few Tequila shots and a half bottle of Jack Daniels, Ezra and I go to the ladies room where we do half a bag of coke in a cubicle and sit on the

DRIPFEED

floor drooling. Ladies come in to use their room; these are not the kind of ladies who will look at Ezra and think, 'what the fuck is a boy doing in this room?' These are the kind of ladies who will look at him, wishing they had a gay best friend as pretty as mine.

Someone wrote 'Blood Controls Everything,' on a Tampax machine in front of me. I am too stoned to appreciate the irony of this, though I can almost taste it, like iron in my mouth.

Someone comes into the toilet; it's Maria, standing by the open door with a weird smile on her face, dangling a small bag of blue and white pills. "Blue or white?" She asks. "Whatever," I say, and she tosses the bag.

Two skinny bitches push past Maria into the body of the toilet. They step over Ezra and me to reapply their eyeliner in mirrors so defaced they might as well be reapplying in the dark. One of the girls doesn't bother with the make-up, she writes something on the mirror instead. I can't see past her to see what she wrote until she leaves.

Maria comes over and sits in the space the skinny bitches have just vacated.

"I'm gonna squeeze you till you squeak." I voice the words the girl wrote on the glass to no one in particular. Then I open the bag and pop two of the pills, both white. I swallow and wait for the shit to happen. When it hits I know it hit. I feel both relaxed and happy at the same time, and I have this overwhelming urge to get up and dance.

Lami Okrekson

Even the sound of the cubicle doors closing is enough to send my feet into Michael Jackson mode.
 Then my brain starts to go completely numb until it bursts out of my head and I go blind without it. I can't feel my head or my body; I can't even hear the sounds of the band playing on the other side of the wall. Sometimes my brain comes back and I see Maria laughing and dancing in front of me, then it is pulled away from me again and it all goes dark.
 Now I am floating up and away from my body, even though I can't see anything I know I'm floating up out of the toilet even. There is no way I could be this weightless and still be on the ground. It's too impossible.

Soon I am back on the ground and the sounds of all those doors closing and all those people talking is just too much for me. I grab Maria and we start dancing crazy wild on the floor. Ezra looks over at us from time to time, too strung out on coke to even notice he's drooling.

DRIPFEED

Chapter 1

Ezra and I have known each other forever. Longer, even, than that. From way back when, when all we did was lie on the grass in Ezra's garden while his parents told us about left wing politics and played 'Purple Haze' and 'Manic Depression.'

Stella liked to move house a lot. Each time she got a bigger promotion at work we'd up sticks and leave; move to a bigger flat, a smaller house, a bigger house. By the time I was eight I felt I had seen enough of London to know I was sick of it. So many bedsits, the insides of so many houses, all mingled together in one collective view of London. Even the cars were changing, as more and more zeroes were added to the end of her bank balance.

I loved the face, the happy one Stella used whenever she broke the good news. 'Another place Cheerio, bigger than this one, with a garden.'

Always her little Cheerio; tiny little O's full of all that wholegrain goodness. Who could resist?

Then Alice's dad came along, and then Alice came along. Then her dad left. And I thought Alice would leave too but she didn't, she stayed with us, so we took her along for the rides as well. Strapped her in the back in a baby seat while I sat up front with Stella, behind the removal vans listening to 'Freak Out' on one of her eighties mix tapes.

One day when I was trapping cockroaches underneath an old jam jar, Stella came into my bedroom. The happy face was on.
"Start packing Cheerio," she said. "We're moving today." Stella was smiling, Alice was in her arms smiling, and I was smiling because they were. I could put all this creepy crawly bullshit behind me now. No cockroaches in the suburbs, I hoped.

It took me an hour to pack. What did *I* have that could have taken any longer? Some clothes and shoes that I shoved into a couple of bin liners. It was the nineties and I didn't have any CD's, just one cassette that had 'My Boy Lollipop' on both sides. Stella stripped my bed, the removal men would take care of all the heavy lifting, but they might get the sheets dirty.
Even though there were only two of us in the house, two real people I mean – Alice didn't count, it seemed the walls were swelling and heaving around us. "Want some Coke, sweetie?" Stella asked.

Riding in the passenger's seat with Stella always made me smile. I felt like she was all mine again, like even Alice's crying couldn't take her away from me. Ha! I felt like shouting at the decrepit old building. We're leaving to go and live in a nice

DRIPFEED

big house in the suburbs, and you're just falling apart.

The car rides were always the best; the eighties funk music tapes, Alice singing along, baby-style, in the back. Driving along, just behind the removal van, watching the houses get bigger and further apart. More trees, driveways, garages; less litter and dog shit on the pavement. The only thing missing from those nineteen fifties throwbacks were the Partridge family and their white picket fence.

We let the removal van go on ahead of us, and drove to the primary school I would be attending. Even the school was perfect, like a mini-Harvard for miniature doctors and lawyers. The building itself was red brick, like every other school in South East London; but it had ivy growing up the sides on some of the walls, and there were huge green fields out towards the back and sides. It was such an improvement on all the other schools I had attended, with their battered footballs and broken gates. Those buildings had looked more like the council estates we were trying to leave behind.

The school, my new school, still had the Boys and Girls signs etched into the concrete above the two main entrances – left over from the Victorian times when this place was built.

There was another gate, a main one in between the two boys and girls' gates. This one had a black grille with a small silver intercom attached. Children filed out from a main door behind this gate in twos, the crocodile, holding hands, their lunch boxes. Even the uniforms were so much cleaner looking, closer to what I wanted than anything I'd ever had. The girls were in blue and white checked pinafores, white polo necks underneath, frilly white socks tucked inside black buckle-up Kickers. The boys were in grey shorts, white polo necks, and long white socks slipping down the insides of muddy, scuffed Hush Puppies. They even looked like the Victorian times, all neatly combed side partings and long sensible braids. Stella looked over at them, imagining me all spruced up in my own checked pinafore and Kickers; holding hands with my own Hush-Puppied boy. How many partners did they even have? We were taught to be loose even then.

Back at the house Stella had cigarettes with the removal men; boys, she called them.

    The house was an actual house this time, none of that Maisonette bullshit where you tell yourself it's really yours, even though you share it with another family. Or flats even, we still referred to those as houses. This house was a house, and it was big, way bigger than anything we'd ever had before. It had a garage and a drive, just like all the rest. Even the neighbours peering through the net curtains at us looked nice.

    As nice as the house was though, it was still another place in another part of London at another time of my life. It was all just a part of the routine. We moved and we moved and we

DRIPFEED

moved. Just another place to take up residence until the annual salary improved and we moved up again. It was inevitable; I knew that even then. I didn't want to grow too attached to that lovely house with the trees and the converted attic, who knew when we'd be back on the road again, behind yet another removal van listening to more retro cassette tapes.

I leant against the side of the car, which was hot considering the day was hot and the engine was still warm, and watched Stella smoking cigarettes and talking to the 'boys.' I fingered one of the cigarettes in my pocket, one I had stolen from the packet on the dashboard, one I would be smoking later, just to see what all the fuss was about. The way Stella and the men kept smoking them, lighting one after another in an endless chain, you'd think they tasted of liquorice and Cherry Drops.

Having kids didn't break the habit then?

Stella saw me watching and dragged me over, pinning me to her side, where the men patted my head and told me what a cute little girl I was; like they hadn't seen me a few hours ago. They oohed and ahhed, Stella joined in too, telling them how intelligent I was for an eight year old, how I always came top of my class.

The day wore on, the removal men did their job, Stella paid them and they went home. Then we went inside to truly look at our house. It was the same as every other house we left behind, filled with all our junk, accumulated over the years that we couldn't just throw in the recycling bin.

I started school the next day. Stella didn't have time to get me a uniform, so I went in my regular clothes instead. I stood out like working class nightmare in amongst all those posh, rich suburban kids.
I saw him right away, tall, floppy black hair, and no front teeth. He was the tallest in the class back then.
      He wasn't wearing the proper uniform either, not when his parents were too laid back to worry about their son conforming to society's warped idea of what a good child *should* look like. He was wearing tie-dyed trousers, brown sandals, and had some brown, African-looking beads around his neck. The beads and his complexion told me he had been on holiday, as did his wild tales of elephant riding and ocean diving later on. Indian beads then. He was a miniature version of his parents, and they loved it. He was free enough to do (and wear) what he wanted, but middle classed enough to not give a fuck. "Hi," he said shaking my hand. "I'm Ezra, who are you?"

DRIPFEED

Chapter 2

"Pass me the needle you fucking whore!"

"Get your own fucking needle," I reply in response to Ezra's command, completely ignoring the fact that he called me a fucking whore. "And didn't they teach you anything in PSE, about not sharing your needles with anyone? What if I've got AIDS?"

Ezra lunges over and wrenches the needle from my arm. I half expect to see a gallon of blood come pouring from there. When I look down my veins will be hanging from my arms, blue and bloodless. When I actually look down there's nothing except the tiny pinprick and a faint scratch.

"If you've got AIDS, I've got AIDS," Ezra sings. "We're all dying anyway so what's the point?"

I'm about to answer him, but the heroin takes me to a happy place where orgasms grow on trees and little blue men hand out strawberry flavoured Vicodin. I take one of the pills from a little man and gradually everything melts together in one hazy, beautiful dream. Ezra singing 'don't share your needles with nobody but me baby,' in the background, even the sound of a lawnmower somewhere downstairs in a garden, seems so far away.

This is a feeling so perfect I want to share it with everyone I know. The slight dizziness could never distract me from the fact that I am completely content with the world. I am wrapped in cotton wool, nothing can harm me now.

Somewhere in between my brush with illicit felicity and the rest of my life, a bell rings. This bell is attached to an elevator, off of which steps a greatly concealed piece of me.

We read about such reunions in 'Hello' magazine, or watch them unravel under the vast wing of Oprah Winfrey or Ricki Lake. In these circumstances, such reunions are joyous affairs where, instead of strawberry flavoured pills, the men bring helium-filled balloons, chocolate muffins and a very appreciative crowd. Appreciative of what exactly? Five minutes of someone else's happiness?

When confronted with this new development, I wish I could say 'thank you,' 'hello' at least. But instead my brain fucks up again and instead of answering the door dressed neatly in Laura Ashley and pearls, I am lying crying in a ball on the floor. It has gotten a hold of me and I don't know how to make it let go.

So my dad is back, again. Ezra and I take walks under the bridge where the skater boys hang. We say nothing about anything. We didn't come here to talk, we didn't even come here to watch skaters trying to impress us with moves they ripped from Tony Hawks 'Proskater.' We came here to be. This is the only place we can truly be without falling off the edge. We are constantly being

DRIPFEED

bitten by the sharks at our feet. They don't ever sleep and we are a generation of insomniacs.

"Ignarus est defaeco of animus," Ezra says.

I don't bother saying 'huh,' or 'what?' I don't even pretend to know what he means. These are things Ezra says when there is nothing else left. We carry on living under Ezra's unanswered question, cry for help; whatever. We carry on towards the edge where the two sides of the coin meet up; the skater boys and the graffiti artists – although 'art' is too pretentious a word to describe their infliction on these crumbling walls. Someone wrote 'Rob woz ere 2001' and I feel like finding Rob and throwing him into the River Thames. If you're going to write something on a wall, at least write something witty. 'Rob woz ere 2001' just doesn't cut it. Dates are overrated anyway, they fade out too quickly.

"So your dad," Ezra says.

"Yeah," I say. This is not why I came here. If I wanted to talk about my dad I would find a psychiatrist. Such things don't need to be discussed; it's like lightning or clouds. No one asks why they are, they just are.

"What does he want?" Ezra will not let go. "Who knows," I say. "Anyway, I didn't really talk to him. Mostly he spoke to Stella about…"

"Yeah." Ezra knows.

"I'll probably see him over the weekend or something," I say. "Get some money out of him."

"Cool." Ezra finally decides to change the subject. "You know I was playing Pokemôn last night."

By now we've left the graffiti and the art and the skater boys. In a minute we'll be back up in the open air, opposite the Hayward, telling ourselves we'll go there one day.

"Pokémon! Isn't that on Nintendo 64 or something?"

"Yeah."

"Oh. I thought the Nintendo 64 was put to sleep at the birth of the Playstation. Now that we're seconds away from Playstation 3, I just assumed all traces of the N64 had been burned in a massive farewell ceremony." My sarcasm doesn't faze Ezra at all.

"Whatever," he says. "It's all about the Nintendo 64. N64's retro like shoulder pads."

"Fuck off," I say. All this talk about games consoles is boring me.

"Come on Puss, it'll only hurt if you let it," Ezra sings to me.

We carry on walking along the bridge to the bus stop, where the water looks all inviting and shit. When I went to the Millennium Dome, in the Millennium, there was this board that had all the different types of fish that live in the Thames on it. I thought that was weird, how fish could survive in all that shit. Even though I know the Thames is filled with the rotting faeces of Ezra's ancestors, I still want to jump in there and disappear for a while. It's just a big headfuck, the growing pains

DRIPFEED

of trying to be a kid in a desperate housewives, middle-classed, wet dream.

"How's Chavez?" Ezra asks.

I don't look at him when he says this, instead I look straight ahead. I know he has raised an eyebrow at the prospect of a lesbian affair. "I looked in the fridge and it was empty," I say. I am actually talking about my fridge at home, which was empty when I left this morning. I wonder if Ezra will get this, or if his hypersensitive imagination will read into things that really aren't there. Ezra is silent and I wonder what he's thinking. We carry on towards the bus stop in silence, with our hands in our pockets. The wind keeps blowing in my face and I can hardly see to walk straight. At times like this I am thankful for the wind, I don't know how Chavez is, nor do I even care. This wind acts as a barrier, between my answer and Ezra's expectation of me. Without it I would be forced to indulge upon his weird little fantasies of what might have been. I haven't seen Maria Chavez since the night in the toilet; it almost seems as if time made a jump cut from then to now, where Ezra still won't let her go.

Sometimes my dad calls, and I jump on double deckers filled with old people smell and the young boys Stella refers to as 'ruff-necked hoodlums.' My dad calls me Pumpkin, which makes me cringe; I'm not used to all that sentimental bullshit. Stella wasn't too ample in the love department and it still feels weird having this stranger call me that.

What is even more strange and weird is when he

tries to hug me. Then, I automatically stiffen. It's as if I don't want the hugs – its always nice at the right time – it's just that hugging a man feels weird, and I still think of him as a stranger.

My dad appears in and out of my life, sometimes he appears around the corner while I'm staggering home from an all-nighter, trying to justify wearing shades in the midst of a storm. These are the times when my abilities as an Oscar-worthy actress are put to the test, and I say things like, I'm fine, nope, haven't found a job yet, but still looking. I say these things whilst trying to balance my hangover on both legs and simultaneously keep my stoned eyes from rolling out of my head.

Then the visits stop, the phone calls become fewer and further between, and I find me spiralling in a downward maelstrom that I would be enjoying were I up to my eyes on some speedball or other.

In other words, I go a bit schizo, just as everyone was expecting anyway. I lock myself in the bathroom with a bottle of Stella's finest vodka and a packet of her most noxious sleeping pills.

Until they start banging on the door, I have no intention of doing anything other than rattling the pills around and causing a bit of unrest for the headfucks on the other side of the door. But now, now that I have their attention, and by 'their' I mean Stella's, something has to happen, otherwise all this was just pointless theatre and wouldn't even get a review in The Mercury.

DRIPFEED

"Charlotte – I mean Chuck, please come out." Stella is pleading through the fucking plasterboard now. As if I'd come out for that, as if the affliction of her wasn't enough, she has to go and humiliate me in front of my friends as well.

"Leave her in there." The sarcastic intonations of Belle creeping under the crack at the bottom of the door, talking about me as if I'm not even there. "She won't do anything with them, come back in a few hours and she'll be asleep on the rug."

Fuck you Belle, for thinking you're better than me, for thinking you even belong in my universe.

"Chuck please!" Stella pleads again.

Then for no reason at all, except that Belle has, once again, tricked me into believing she was my friend and wormed her way into my house, I get really, really pissed off. Worse than before, if I was schizo before, I am truly fucking psychotic now. This is the real fucking deal and I'm going to see it through to the end.

"Fuck off!" I say. "I have a monster headache and I'm just gonna take a couple of these pills to kill the pain and go to sleep for a while."

"Chuck no!" Stella is wailing now, as if that's going to make a difference. And in that instance, I truly hate her. I can almost see her through the wood, going through her usual overdose routine; hunched over on all fours, mascara dripping down cheeks whilst Ezra pats her on the back, not really caring but doing it because no one else will.

I pour the entire bottle on the floor, it'll look better this way, when they finally break through all that wood and find me lying here, lifeless and blue on the matching aquatic rug. I take the pills in huge handfuls, swallowing some with the vodka and some dry – because the vodka makes me retch and I can't afford for this not to work.

If this was an attention-seeking stunt before, I am pretty fucking serious now.

Somewhere underneath my psychosis, I actually believe that I have a headache, and I'm just doing all this to relieve it and get some sleep. But closer to the surface where I really am, I really want to die.

I'm getting a bit hazy from all the pills now and everything is starting to go all soft and fuzzy round the edges. Even my brain feels like it's encased in cotton wool. I know I'm drowning now, but it doesn't hurt like the other times, they felt like an elephant stampede in my head. This feels like dying, but it feels too nice to hurt.

Stella is still wailing outside and I manage to take another half-sip of vodka before shouting, "You should have paid more attention Stella, then maybe Timmy wouldn't be so dead right now."

There is a pause before Stella's belated reply rebounds off the wooden door. "Who's Timmy?" she asks.

DRIPFEED

I take another sip, which is making me stronger, bolder somehow, like I'm stronger even than the little white pills on the rug. "It doesn't matter. Timmy's dead and you could have saved him if you paid more fucking attention."

"Chuck!"

"Chuck's not here," I say. "Chuck's gone on a fucking hiatus. Didn't you see the 'gone fishing' sign on the door? There's nobody home."

Then I go for another handful of pills, but there's only one left and I need that for them. So I try to stand up instead, thinking that if this shit isn't going to work I might as well open the door and let them in. I think I get the door open; I can't be sure, because when I sit up, time made another jump cut. Instead of lying with my head busted open on the ceramic tiles, four men are holding me down whilst another shoves a tube down my throat. They keep telling me to swallow the tube and I don't know how they expect me to do that. Women dressed in white, who vaguely resemble milk bottles, appear from nowhere bearing polystyrene bowls. I throw up in the bowls and then people are wiping my head and telling me I'm going to make it; this time.

I don't want to make it.

"Are you okay?" Ezra asks. "Because that was some serious shit. This isn't Girl Interrupted you know. There's only so many times you can OD without dying."

Lami Okrekson

Funny how he's all concerned about me now, when it really counts, but he'll still ply me with all this shit anyway. If only we were flight attendants, then we'd be able to get high on oxygen instead of all this man made crap. The little blue men slip in and out of my peripheral and I get ready to pick an orgasm off of a tree.

Chavez is here too, so are Charlie and Belle. They passed out ages ago though, if this were my house, I'd kick them onto the lawn and make them sleep off their hangovers outside.

Chavez stares at me for the whole night. Even when I'm asleep, I dream I'm awake and she's still staring at me. When I am awake we have nothing to say to each other, we just lay there with needles hanging out of our arms and tongues hanging out of our heads.

I start having dreams about lips; huge red lips attacking me from all angles. These are soundless, terrifying dreams that leave me waking up drenched in sweat. It's not the fact that the lips are attacking, it's that they don't seem to be attached to bodies, they just float above me, soundlessly attacking me with their flesh. Sometimes they stay with me for hours after I wake, I think I see them in the mirror, or etched into a wall somewhere, taunting me wordlessly. I would never scream out like they do in the movies, I could never be so abject. Girls who wake from nightmares screaming annoy me. I don't

DRIPFEED

understand why they can't just turn the light on and forget about it like I do.

Chapter 3

Ezra tells me about the first time his parents gave him an e.
"Why'd they give you an e?" I ask.
"I dunno," he says. "They just did."
I don't question this, whether or not it is true, Ezra has those kinds of parents, the ones who don't mind if you do a little experimenting in your youth, 'as long as you don't get hooked mind,' never get hooked. God forbid you end up in rehab.

We are sitting on the grass at our school, outside the building, where all the scenesters hang, smoking their skinny, multi coloured cigarettes and talk about their fictitious bouts with depression and rehab. Any minute now they're all going to start crying into their coffee about their drunken mummies on the couch. Emos cry about everything. If they're so emotional then maybe they shouldn't wear so much mascara.
Some of our teachers are here also, on the grass smoking their cigarettes and drinking tea from polystyrene cups. Probably they are talking about how much they'd like to run us over with their cars, how much we piss them off and all that. From here we can see everything. Ezra finishes one Marlboro, stubbing it out on the grass and lighting up a fresh one.
"Why did the referee throw the watch?" He asks. He's reading off of the back of a bag of

DRIPFEED

Wotsits, the kind with the really shitty jokes on the back that are supposed to have kids rolling on the grass clutching their sides to keep their insides in.

"I don't know," I say. "Why did the referee throw the watch?"

"To see time fly," Ezra says without laughing.

I take another cigarette from the packet on the grass between us. Today is one of the rare days in June where we are blessed with twenty degrees and a whole lot of sun. Despite the sun, and the grass, and the anorexic dancers prancing around in less than their leotards, the emos are still wearing their skinny black jeans and big woollen cardigans. They need all that wool to soak up their tears.

"Remember when we first met Chavez and she gave you those pills?" Ezra asks.

"No," I say.

"Yeah you do," Ezra pushes. "She gave them to you so you would loosen up. You know she likes you."

It's a statement rather than a question and the only thing I can think of to say is, "Whatever."

"Wanna go see Madonna in concert?" Ezra says.

I close my eyes and red, bodiless lips float behind my closed lids. Faint smells of Formaldehyde and blood sink up through the grass and into my atmosphere. These smells bring with them waves of nostalgia I can't place.

Lami Okrekson

The last day of school comes and goes without a bang, except we eat Hula Hoops, drink Coca Cola from polystyrene cups and pretend to be entertained by funk music from the eighties. Our teachers prance around, drunk off their own excitement, and the emos cry into their black handkerchiefs by the door. Then there's the wannabes, the ones walking around outside looking like they're wearing someone else's clothes and trying too hard to look cool. They try and creep into our photographs and smoke stolen cigarettes outside of the emos, far enough not to be guilty by association, but close enough to feel the waves of them like an electric undercurrent.

After the Coke is finished, and the polystyrene cups have been cleared away, the photographs taken and the leavers' books written in, someone suggests Pizza, so we pile into cars and end up outside a Pizza Hut somewhere.

After Pizza Hut we end up at a party where we drink Sambuca straight from the bottle. I end up drinking more than anyone else, more than Ezra even and end up passing out with my head in a toilet. I wake up later, at five a.m. on a couch, I have no idea how I made it here and what happened to my coat - which is in a pile on the floor with my shoes.

I get up and follow the sounds of my peers, who are lying on three beds that have been pushed together to make one huge bed. I crawl in amid them, and fall asleep to the stories of what I did before I passed out.

DRIPFEED

We go back to school for exams, and I'm too ashamed to say anything. Everyone obviously knows what happened, they're just too afraid to antagonise me - who knows what I got up to that night. They carry on as normal, as before, with their leaver's books and their cameras.

The cameras, the fucking cameras, all this shit in my face. Didn't we get all this out of our systems last time? They all want a piece of me; they've all set out to put me under the spotlight in front of the fucking lens.

Chavez comes back and it's like she never left. She's here now, on the outside of my wardrobe while I'm inside crying again. I have visions of people hanging by their necks from helium-filled balloons; floating over central London's corporate step ladders. Somewhere off to the side of them, men wait on top of a building - maybe Canary Wharf - waiting to jump. They take turns in jumping soundlessly over the edge. Each time one jumps, another one is added to the end of the queue. What happens to these men after they jump is beyond me, I don't follow them that far down. In my deluded, fucked-up world, we land on pillowcases filled with blue flowers and the corners of tin foil. Perhaps that's where these men will end up too.

Alice is here too, in her eleven year old skin, cutting things out of a Littlewoods magazine - she ran out of Argos magazines. There are going to be cut-up bits of paper all over my room when I get out of here, but this doesn't piss me off as much as it usually would have. In fact, it doesn't piss me off at all.

"Want some crystal baby?" Chavez asks me.

"No!" I scream. "Give me some fucking coke!"

"I got some poppers from that sex shop on Tottenham Court road," she supplies without prompting.

"So?"

"So do you want some? I haven't done poppers for ages." I don't have time for this bullshit. Poppers are shit; they don't even last long enough to feel. Poppers are for eleven year old sociopaths like Alice. I'm about to join the queue behind the men on top of Canary Wharf.

"I said give me some fucking coke Chaz!"

"Relax baby," Chavez says. "It's coming." She pushes a little clear plastic bag underneath the door. I don't even want it anymore; I don't want any of it. I close my eyes and jump off of the building, except I don't land in the pillowcases, I don't land on anything. I try to open my eyes and look for me, but I'm lost. Maybe I really have gone fishing, who even knows anymore?

I decided that God deserted me a long time ago; prayed for a better life, a better mother, all the things we are entitled to. "But God loves everyone," they said. Bullshit! If He loves everyone then why doesn't He love me? I've just decided that heaven is not where I'll be. Unless

DRIPFEED

I'm thrown back to earth and given a second chance as a praying mantis or a flower, then I'm going straight to hell. That's what the evangelists tell me anyway, they see through my eyes into the sin lurking beneath my soul.

I'd be a child again if I could. If I could just get to eleven and stop, and repeat the whole process again. Your only responsibilities as a child are keeping your nose clean and your shoelaces tied up properly. Then you become an adult and responsibility hits like acid rain. We could say, life sucks, but that'd be a cliché.

Thankfully, I'm not yet at that age where the reins are handed over to me and I am forced to superintend my whole life. I'm allowed to be here, for now, as this cartoon image of myself, though I did not see it coming.

Feminist English teachers taught us to be shrewd, to look beneath the surface for what, at first, seems invisible. And it worked, we became manipulative and vindictive. So how come we don't see the blood gushing out of our own open scar tissue? How come we failed to register the pain at the point of entry? What happened?

I realise I must have slit my wrists again because there's blood on the floor and it's coming from me. It's fascinatingly petrifying and awesome as well. The blood looks pretty running down my arms and the little pools collecting on the floor dilate like pupils.

I try to bite back the urge to deface; anything. It is stronger than I am but thankfully I resist. Or rather, I am too stoned and too dead to will my limbs out of useless entropy and do anything with them. I am, however, strong enough to take another hit in veins that are already bleeding me to death.

Then things start to happen; Chavez calls for Stella, who sends sociopath Al up instead. Then of course she follows suit - I am not important enough to drag her away from her Eastenders. She's seen it all before anyhow, me on the floor, locked inside something with blood seeping through the cracks at the bottom. How many times does she need to see me like this before she realises that there is a problem?

Stella takes her time getting here; maybe she wants me to kill myself. If this doesn't work I'll be forced to do it some way that seems accidental; like accidentally leaving the gas on and sealing all exists, or forgetting to look both ways at the intersection. She'd never know she won. It's never about taking part with her, and she'd die of the humiliation.

When we finally make it to the emergency room, where I'm bleeding about a pint a minute and the nurses are all tut-tutting as they remember me from last time, I wonder what happened to the cocaine in the bag on the floor of the wardrobe, and how, even though I've just slashed my wrists, I feel like I've taken four lithium tablets. A silent victory, until the doctors whack another tube down my throat, assuming I've OD'd on pills again - I am a regular here it seems.

DRIPFEED

    Then it's over, and there's wires coming out of my head, and wires going into my hands, and Stella's by my bed screaming in her head and trying to let the nurses see the tears she's crying. "Oh Charlotte," she says.
    "It's Chuck, you fucking bitch!"

There was a time before, before I hated Stella, before someone said, 'want me to go get some coke?' Before 'coke' meant cocaine and no one knew what cigarettes tasted like. Funnily enough, the 'before' is where all this shit should have started, where the skin heads sat shooting up on decaying staircases that should have been derelict. In retrospect, she hated me even then; she must have, because everything I know about her has been regurgitated to me from someone else's gut. Because I know nothing about her, or him, or how they even met, I have to make it up. In my head I have my ideas of how they met, when they met, where.

Since Stella was pushing twenty-five, husband and child-less, she would have thrown herself at the first man to say hello. So I presume they met at a Valium factory, where they were both stocking up on their monthly supply. She would have been on her way in while he was coming out; their eyes would have met over little brown bottles of little tiny pills. Then what? Who knows, I haven't fabricated that much. All I know is that after they had me he left. She and I were never close enough for her to divulge the finer details.

But after that, the regular memories come flooding back, walks home from Sunday school, Stella looking all pretty and nice-smelling (probably trying to trap another man with her poison ivy lasso). People telling me how young and pretty she was how lucky I was to be hers, and not the property of some part-time prossie from the estate.

It's kind of funny, how most kids from divorced families at least have early memories of their fathers - waking up, going to sleep, feeding them pieces of mashed-up apple with the skin taken off - and yet I have none. Not even a smile or a smell to remind me of anything. This is why he came as a complete shock to me in ninety-three. Strangely enough, I don't even know if he's changed between then and now. When it comes to my father I have the memory of a goldfish.

Growing up on a council estate had its perks, close-knit neighbourhood - about as close to Desperate Housewives as you're going to get in south-east London's ghetto slums. I like to believe though, that it contributed in some way to me now. As though the staircase crack whores and skinhead junkies I never saw somehow filtered into my subconscious and stuck, like pinecones, to my frontal lobe. That shit wasn't glamorised, it didn't even look comfortable; all hunched over like that, with ten-inch hypodermics shoved into bulging green veins.

DRIPFEED

Those were my friends though, and that was my playground, amid the used needles, pretending not to know what they were for. Or collecting snails in little plastic bags, watching them slime their way across each other, trying to find a way out, eventually sliming themselves to death.

It was fun; at least it was the only fun we knew. It was beautiful, huge and entertaining; but smaller somehow, depressing even, when I go past it on the train now. It hasn't changed, I haven't even changed, I just got taller and saw it from a new angle.

Stella doesn't creep into these memories, but I know she was there.

I am lying on my bed listening to *Exit…music for a film* on a loop when Ezra calls.

"What's the problem?" he asks.

What is the problem? More to the point, what is *the* problem? What is it now that could be so fucking debilitating - and the 'now' is a huge part of it - that all I want to do is lie here in the dark with the curtains closed? I am lacking, even, in the ability to get up and brush my teeth. This little act of defiance isn't hurting anyone but me. *I'm* the one who will have to endure the cavities and the plaque, the pain of having them filled in by trigger-happy dentists. So why don't I just get up and brush like a normal person?

It's not just *my* life that is a series of events, it's life in general. Every up, every down, every sideways turn, is just an event in a long, monotonous series. And these events are never new, they never change, namely, we are never surprised. Life goes round and round and round. The same red car passes by three times in one hour; the same baby is always at the station, crying when you need some quiet time to ease the inner voices into oblivion.

There must be someone, somewhere, pulling all these strings, giving the directions, pinching the babies to make them cry. All of this cannot be chance, on the off chance I'm at the library for some quiet time, the same punk in the same green t-shirt is there, giving me the same looks, sitting in the same fucking chair. It's all too much of a coincidence to be coincidence; too predictable.

Even the librarians don't say hello anymore.

This brings me back to my problem, me trying to find out what is wrong with me now, what changed between here and then that made such a huge impact. It must have been a series of events; surely I would have noticed if it were one single one, I would have felt something click at the exact moment my life changed.

It has something to do with the world, this much I know. Or rather, the way the world is so against me. Everyone knows something about me; some deep, dark secret I thought was safe in my head, something they will all use against me when the time is right. I can't shake this paranoia, that's what it is, crazy, stupid, meaningless rubbish. But how else do I explain it? The looks,

DRIPFEED

everyone looking. Always looking at me. I walk into a room and all eyes are on me, bend over to pick up a pen and - oh yeah! - all eyes are on me.

I know what's going on. This is the huge conspiracy theory they warned us about. The Truman Show, Nineteen Eighty-Four, Big – fucking – Brother. All of them are Big Brother and they're all watching. Me. Constantly watching me all the time. The weird thing is though, if this is the conspiracy theory, why aren't they hiding it better? Why are they so fucking obvious? They don't try to conceal the looks they give me. These aren't even looks that could be put down as sly. These are full-on, bang in my face, frontal stares. They stare like they've never seen people before. Like I'm some kind of E.B.E or something. Some ancient throw-back to Roswell.

"Maybe they're attracted to you," someone suggested once. Or not. Maybe they know. Maybe they saw me on television last night, smoking that green.

But wouldn't you have seen it?

No! Because they know. They know when I'm about to change the channel and they change. Everyone knows, it's not a secret. Stella's probably in on it too, maybe that's why she's such a bitch to me all the time, because it makes for good television. They all want a piece of me, to put in their time capsules to the year 2050. Why can't they just leave it alone? Leave me alone! I'm nothing special; there are more fucked-up people than me out there. Why me? Out of all the billions of other people in the world, people who eat other people, people who have three legs, four arms, five eyes - why me!?

What have I done to deserve this shit?

"Why did you run off like that?" Ezra asks.

We were in Camden; Ezra was getting a tattoo in this dark, hardcore place by the loch. Belle and Charlie were there too. Belle picked up a neon pink lighter from a basket - the kind that glows in the dark and lights up when you light up.

"Yo Chuck!" she called. "This would look good on you." She tossed it to me. It was still hot from where she had been trying it out.

Belle is sarcastic to the core. She wasn't being nice, suggesting I splash out on this 99p lighter to be kind. Pink has never been my colour, and as for pretty, glow-in-the-dark lighters, what the fuck? Fuck that! I don't want something that draws so much attention to me. I'm happy to light my cigarettes off candles or matches. Who needs all this pink shit when it amounts to the same thing in the end? A lit cigarette. A stick that burns. Burnt paper and tobacco. Why bother?

I bought the lighter anyway, matches aren't so good for cooking with, and they burn out too quickly against the metal. Holding a match upright for too long burns your fingertips - and you can hardly turn the spoon upside down. I bought the lighter and Belle was happy because she made me do something I really didn't want to do. I didn't need it; we already established that - it won't even

DRIPFEED

look good on my table. Red's my thing, red Marlboros, red match box, and a red t-shirt. Pink just doesn't fit in there, in amongst all that red; inside a snooker club, hitting red and yellow balls around a green table. Pink is too contrasting; it clashes with all the other colours of my life.

I didn't even use the lighter right away. I went back outside the shop to light a cig, I even asked some guy to borrow his lighter. He looked at the neon pink one in my hand and shrugged. He gave me his cigarette; he didn't have time for rummaging around in his rucksack for his own lighter. No one has time for that, if they do it's because they're desperate. They need that distraction from themselves, and you're the only one who can give it to them.
 The man was gone by the time I looked up; he wasn't even visible amongst the throng of people that surged forward to conceal him from me. Maybe he wasn't one of them; maybe he was one of me. They knew it, they always do. They had to get rid of the problem before I found out too much.

I finished the cigarette and went back inside, downstairs, to where the branding was taking place.
 Downstairs was such a contrast to upstairs. Upstairs was so dark, so weird and gothic, downstairs was bright like TK Maxx. It was so bright I had to put my shades on. It wasn't like outside, where the only light comes from the sun

so you don't have to look at it. This was pure, distilled, artificial decadence. It came from everywhere, the floors, the ceilings, even the walls. Too many lights showing up too many of my imperfections. I need to keep some things for myself.

It wasn't the lights that got to me in the end, it was the sound. So mechanical, so damaging. The light showed every detail of Ezra's face as that sharp, mechanical needle ripped into his arm. The forearm. It was a surprise they even agreed to do it. But then *tattoo* is to junky what *baggy jumper* is to the obese. It conceals that scar tissue we want to keep for ourselves.

    I don't know why Ezra was grimacing the way he was, its not like he didn't have time to get used to needles, we all did.

    The man doing the tattoo looked like a giant. That's all I can say. He looked, like a giant. Big matted beard, bushy eyebrows, deep voice, extra pounds, covered in tattoos. The kind of trailer-trash neo-goth you see on Ricki Lake. The red-neck hillbillies, pawning their grandmother's cha cha for a new motorbike. He looked like a trucker from a film about truckers, the kind who frequent diners and bars that have 'truckers only' signs on the door. If he were pinning me to a bench with a needle, I'd be grimacing too. If he had me dissected like that I don't know if I'd be able to stay there. I'd be up on the bench demanding to be anaesthetised. Or, I'd be out the door, with half a tattoo, running as fast as I could.

DRIPFEED

That's what I did, when it all got too much; the lights, the mechanical 'wurr' of the needle, the giant and his beard, the neon pink lighter glowing in the dark of my pocket.

I must have experienced some kind of hysterical fugue, because then I was back home, lying on my bed, listening to Radiohead. I had no recollection of the train rides home, of even getting from the tattoo parlour – what a word – to the station. My memory took a break and joined me in my bed later for a cigarette and a song.

"Well?" Ezra prompts. The neon pink lighter is here with me now, on the table so, although the curtains are closed, it's not glowing. These curtains don't block out enough of the light to satisfy me. What I want is a pair of black velveteen curtains that are allowed to envelope me in complete silence. I like the lighter now; it was there to experience the fugue with me. I use it to light the cigarette and drag deeply before answering. Which question though? Which question shall I answer first? First of all, I do not know what the problem is. I thought I did but I don't. That or it's too big to explain. And it isn't just one problem, it's a series of tiny little ones, and it would take too long to dissect. I'd be here all day just trying to think up a way to explain the first.

"It was too bright in there,"

"So why didn't you say? Why did you just leave like that?" I don't know. I really do not have the answers to all these questions. I don't even have the energy for this conversation. I want to hang up and smoke my way through the next twelve runs of this song. "Is that Radiohead in the background?" Ezra asks. More questions. Adding more and more questions to the list. Questions upon questions upon lists upon lists of bullshit. I can't handle. This.

I press 'cancel' on the phone and switch it off. I'm still nervous and jittery from all those lights, all that noise, all those people in my face. The only one who really understands me and how I feel is the lighter. The neon pink lighter on the table next to my bed is the only thing on this earth that really and truly understands what it is I am going through at this minute. The lighter. Neon pink. Picked out for me by Belle, my archenemy. Silver lining and all that crap. She just didn't know.

Now I am deflated. Now I feel like I've been shrink-wrapped. I'm still me but lesser somehow. Some bits of me have been sucked out in a timeless vacuum. I am for sale. I will be shipped overseas in the morning.

It's funny how almost anything can be discovered through 'process of elimination.' The only process sure to reveal. This process though, is long and drawn out. It takes days, sometimes months; years even, to eliminate all possibilities. By eliminating what the problem *isn't*, surely I'll be able to find what the problem *is.* Except, and here's the funny bit, it doesn't work for me. Because everything is the problem. Every

DRIPFEED

molecule, every atom, every element on the periodic table, led me here and added to the new, lesser, me. Trying to decide what the problem *isn't* is almost as hard as trying to decide what the problem *is.*

It's all so tiring. Not just legs aching, eyes drooping, kind of tiring. This is real fatigue. The kind where every bone, every muscle, every cell of your body is so drained, so wasted, that mere sleep isn't enough. Simply lying down in bed just can't cure this tiredness.

Too tired to sleep.

I lay awake instead. Too tired to think, look, *do* anything but breathe. This consumes me, like the shrink-wrap. It is this lack of breathable air that I can't handle. Once again I bit off more than I could chew. Stood up too quickly and received a thousand head rushes at once. Or sat down for too long and found my bum had gone to sleep. How do you wake your arse up when it's just *that* tired?

I stop trying to figure out what's wrong. I'll be fine in the morning. All this is just another phase, like the hula-hoop, or bell-bottoms. I'll get suckered in, I'll be consumed, and then it'll pass. I always ride these things out to the very end.

Belle calls me asking if I'll go with her to some club or other. I say yes. I say this because I am a pushover and 'yes' is what pushovers like me say. I know I won't go, even before the question is out of Belle's mouth, I don't want to. I don't like Belle, and she doesn't like me. In fact, the only reason she asked me to go in the first place was probably because she'd exhausted all other ties. I'm the only one left in her long list of people to spend a Friday night with.

The worst thing about this is not the fact that I said yes, it's that I said 'definitely,' which leaves the presumption that I will be waiting for her at some train station or other, on time. Of course I text her later saying I'm sorry but I really can't... I'm good at that, letting people down I mean, blowing people off. The epitaph on my tombstone will read, 'Charlotte Brown, outstanding wit, excellent dress sense, but undeniable let down.'

I feel bad for a while, as I always do when I feel like I've made someone else feel bad. In truth, Belle probably couldn't care less since she doesn't like me either. She probably found someone else, someone she likes even less, to go with her tonight. But for a while, I watch 'Girl Interrupted!' and try to convince myself that I'm crazy enough to be carted off to some mental health institute for a well-earned rest. I have all the requirements: suicide attempt that resulted in wrist-stitching *and* stomach pumping, tendency to over indulge on the class A's, and frequent bouts with inner demons. Then I look closer, between the black lines; some secret little underground society for the insane, I do not want to be institutionalised.

In truth, I probably don't even qualify for all that shit; I'm not crazy enough. There are no

DRIPFEED

voices inside my head, except my own; which, in some ways is even worse; it's my own voice telling me I'm worthless. This inner, secretive, voice is strong enough to block out Thom Yorke's.

I lie curled up on the floor – wishing I could curl up into someone else's life – listening to Radiohead through earphones, because Stella doesn't like the noise. You would have thought her dreams of perpetual silence would be somewhat shattered by the arrival of children.

      I could go and see a shrink, but they'd only ask what everyone else asks. What is the problem? And I'd get defensive as fuck and say, 'you're the shrink, right? You've had thousands of boys and girls forced onto this couch by despairing mummies and daddies, displaying their wounds and their overdoses. Staring at the walls through dull, listless eyes, lackadaisical bodies slumped across the expansive leather. "I don't know what the problem is. You're the psychiatrist, you tell me." Only I do know what's wrong, and it can't be cured by talk and therapy. It's not depression, it's her.

I overhear her talking about me with Alice, saying I'm in a bad mood because she took the music away, that she doesn't care that I don't care. Alice responding as best as her eleven year old brain will allow, saying all I do is sleep and then wake up angry. Stella saying sleeping all day is bad for me.

Lami Okrekson

So now I've become someone else's case study, something for mother and daughter to discuss over dinner, a dinner, might I add, that I am not invited to. She thinks she knows what's wrong, that I'm having a histrionic because she confiscated my life, not bothering to look closer, at herself. How dare she try and psychoanalyse my problem when she is the only problem!

I try not to think about depression, try and pretend that I don't spend my days curled up in a ball on the floor listening to Radiohead through earphones. Or slicing my arms and legs with Bic razorblades I bought from the chemist. I have no desire to harm my body, unless it promises to get me away from this permanently.

What I have cannot be reconciled by pathological scar tissue. I can't seek pleasure in the opening and closing of wounds because it is not enough. It's too distracting, and I can't afford to be distracted, not when last time I ended up in the emergency room leaking blood from severed wrists.

That was the point where pain hit true and concise, and even through I tried not to, I knew it was the beginning of some new, stationary form of existence.

It is almost funny how people always OD on sleeping pills and antihistamines in the boat ride leading up to wrist slitting and cocaine abuse. Wrist slitting is for wimps, we always know someone is waiting just outside the door to dial

DRIPFEED

999, or that we didn't cut deep enough for any real damage. There are other, more effective ways to commit suicide. For example, hanging or a Valium overdose. These are pleasant ways to go, relax and let the rope do what it has to; even the pills wrap you in a nice security blanket before piercing an already black heart with poison ivy razorblades.

So one day when I was fourteen and Stella's bullshit became too much for me to handle, I went for the only thing I had, my five milligram Levocetirizine Dihydrochloride antihistamines. In retrospect, I kind of knew I wouldn't die; it was more of a cry for help than an actual attempt on my life. I wanted Stella to come in and find me zonked out on the floor, still clutching the little box that once held the tiny white ovals.

I only had seven left, so I popped them all, wrote a brief suicide note, which I left to Alice instructing her to give to Stella should I not wake up. Then I lay down on my bed and went to sleep. Antihistamines are drowsy like that, so it's understandable that I thought I was actually dying as I drifted off.

Then the time between the 'okay times' got longer and longer, and someone said, 'why bother?' and I agreed. I must have passed out then, because I woke up four years later with a pair of scissors in my wrist and a needle in my arm. Who said life was a bitch? We are our own twelve inch cocks and we fuck ourselves in the arse.

Lami Okrekson

I see Ezra again. We take trips down memory lane down Waterloo Bridge and to the lair of the stoners, now abandoned by the crack-whore trick babies. We stand here for a while, while we wait for Belle and Charlie to get down here. Then they arrive, so it's off to the pub where we drown ourselves in alcohol and sing songs about drunken sailors and camels called Alice. It stinks of thrown-up beer, bitter disappointment and bloody Sundays, but none of that matters because the booze is cheap and they don't ID at the door.

I ask Ezra if he remembers secondary school, when we used to bunk – me from my girls' school and him from his boys' school – with an older girl who was still young enough not to have been hit by puberty. We would drink Hooch and run barefoot across some lake, then we would sit on the bank and she would tell us about sex and drugs while we smoked cigarettes she'd bought with fake ID. We knew it was wrong and stupid; we were sharp enough to know a secondary education was important in a world of drunken, depressed, alcoholic mothers and general hereditary fuck-ups. We needed those educations to break the chain of generations failed by their own stupidity, and we knew it, we were just having too much fun to get off our arses and do something about it.

It is World Cup season and there is an important match on. I have no idea whose turn it is. To be honest, I couldn't care less. As far as I'm

DRIPFEED

concerned, it's just a bunch of men chasing a piece of leather up and down a lawn. Besides, it's too violent and bloody, if I wanted to watch men break their bones, I'd stay home and watch ER. None of our group are much interested by the antics on the large flat-screen, we just came for the beer and the crisps, nothing added, nothing taken away.

Belle and Charlie and Ezra and I sit in silence, although the only silence is our own considering we are surrounded by a pub-full of sweaty men yelling insults at athletes for whom they harbour the most intense and damaging jealousy.

When I told Stella I was going out today she sneered and asked what time I'd be back. "I don't know," I said. "Twelve, one?" Stella had sneered again and said, "One? What kind of a pub closes at one? So you're going to stay till the end, I presume, and be the last one to leave like you always are!" I didn't even warrant that remark with a reply. I walked calmly away like the bible taught us to when we still believed in God. I turned the other cheek, became the bigger person, and walked away.

"How's the life?" Ezra asks through a mouthful of smoke.

"Same as ever," I reply. I don't know when Ezra and I became the kind of people who asked each other how life was. The kind of people we hate, like people who own rats, or old ladies who wear fur coats in the middle of July. Somewhere between then and now we drifted. Though Ezra is my only link between sanity and insanity. We are each other's psychiatrists; we needed each other, until now, where we can hardly get past the small talk. He's probably fed up with me, and I don't blame him. I'm fed up with me, tired of stepping outside of myself to watch me break down again.

"You can't keep breaking down every time someone calls you crazy," Ezra says. "Everyone's crazy, so consider it a compliment. You're normal." So we sit, in silence, watching men watching men playing football.

The match is a bore; it drags on for extra time when neither team has scored by the ninetieth minute. I can't help wondering if both teams are equally good, or if they're equally shit. Eventually, we go and sit outside with our pints of beer, where the sun is so hot I can feel my pores opening and closing even though I am sitting still. It's at times like these when I wish I had some weed, or some coke, anything to get me away from the heat of this place.

So Ezra and I leave without telling Charlie or Belle. They won't mind anyway, they're too wrapped up in their own morose lethargy to notice anything.

"When was the last time we went out?" Ezra asks me.

"Dunno," I say. "Feels like ages."

"Yeah," says Ezra, because he always has to get the last word in.

DRIPFEED

Then I say, "Where'd you wanna go?" because I'm the kind of person who feels the need to fill every silence. Silence isn't golden, it's unnerving. You can hear too much in silence, things you don't want to hear, things that would scare the shit out of you if you were in a dark room by yourself.

"Home," says Ezra. "I got some coke last night, we'll have a party."

By the time we get on the tube at Waterloo it's already after nine and I know my bitch mum will have a cow if I'm too late. The coke is temptation enough to disobey her, but for some reason I know not to push it. Not since the informal sleepover, even though that was ages ago.

"I can't come to yours actually," I tell Ezra. "I have to get home."

"Why do you listen to her? I mean, she's cool and everything, but she's a bit crazy like. Why don't you just tell her to fuck off and leave you alone?"

"Cos she'd break my face. She's cool enough when you lot are there, but when it's just me, her and Alice, she goes all psycho bitch."

We stand squashed against the doors of the tube. It's so silent I can hear the cogs turning in my head; I can even hear the rats chewing at the wiring underneath the train. I need to fill this silence. "Why don't you just come to mine?" Even as I ask the question, even as the words come out of my mouth, I want to take them back. I don't want Ezra in my house. I don't want anyone in my house except for me. I am relieved when Ezra says,

"That means going to mine and then yours. That's bare long. I'll call you tomorrow; we'll get fucked up at my cottage."

When I finally get home at ten thirty, I remember I haven't done my chores. Fuck it, I think, I'll do them tomorrow. I go to bed without sleeping; I just lay there, with the window open, staring at the foam squares. It is hotter than the sun in here. Too hot to move. I'd probably sweat to death if I even got up to adjust the covers, which are steadily burning my legs to death. I would like to close the window; the prospect of waking up with a spider on my face is not very pleasant. But to close the window I'd have to get up, I'd have to move, and it's way too hot for any of that. Besides, I just can't be bothered.

I must have fallen asleep then, because the next thing I know it's four a.m. and Stella's waking me up with the bright lights and the commands. Telling me to get up and clean the house, which I do, and then go back to bed tired but not sleeping. She comes in again then, pissed off because I'm not. "What you have failed to do now, I'll wake you up in the middle of the night to do tomorrow," she yells at me before storming out leaving the door open.

I can't help thinking it pointless. What is the point of her? Why can't she just leave me alone? Get a life, get some friends, get out of my face. It's always take, take, take with her. 'What *you*

DRIPFEED

have failed to do! Get up...clean this...wash that,' then put on a clean fucking t-shirt and play nice for the neighbours. Appearance is everything, and we appear to be fine.

I suppose it never occurred to her for one minute, to get down on *her* hands and fucking knees and clean her own shit up. I tried to be indifferent, tried not to care, but all I can do is care and all I can do is hate. And once again I find myself wishing her dead, consumed with rage because she isn't even good at the one thing that should come naturally to her. Once again the same statement resonates like a mantra inside my head, 'if you don't like people, don't have children.' Or, just don't take your fucking psychosis out on the ones you're supposed to be nurturing.

It's funny, how one sentence can pack such a punch that it remains in your head forever, and you know nothing you or anyone will ever say or do can shake it off. Sharks don't sleep so why do we? If I could stay awake through this it might make it more bearable. Sleep only confuses me, provides me with a momentary lapse from myself. But then of course, she's always standing over me, ready to wake me up again; and I don't even know what I've done wrong.

I can't help hating rich, middle-class girls who claim depression like diamond rings. Sit in the bathtub listening to the Velvet Underground, slicing at their legs with the edges of mummy's diamonds or daddy's Gillette. How can these bitches be depressed when they have everything?

Half of them can't even find a tangible source at which to vent their inverted anger. At least I know what's wrong with me. At least I have a fucking excuse, a prelude, a back-story.

I'm five foot four and a half. Five foot fucking four and a half. Always that half-inch away from everywhere. Half an inch away from being adequate, being socially fucking acceptable. It's like I could see what I was going for and I just missed. Shit! Or like the Marlovian Over reacher; reached too far and fell over. Always almost, never fucking there. My nails are too short, or I'm too short. My feet are too big, my jeans are too tight, or they're not tight enough. My belt was too long then I cut it, so now it's too short and I'm stuck because there's nothing I can do about it.

I start to think that maybe this is where all the shit started, where I became the topic of conversation over microwaved chicken curries. If I'd just been five foot five then none of this would have happened. I'd be okay. I'm not exceptional, and that's the problem. I'm not even average; I'm half and inch away from average.

Then Stella comes in, twenty-four hours later, waking me up at two in the morning to bring my clothes in off the washing line. This is just an excuse, since she pretty much told me she was going to wake me up again yesterday. She probably just couldn't find anything else for me to clean. So here I am, at two in the morning, getting my clothes off the hanger, because once again she wants, or doesn't want. She, she, she, she,

DRIPFEED

she. For fucks sake. Yada, yada, yada. Same old fucking line. She has a bad day and decides to let me know about it. She could have just asked me to do it when she realised at ten or eleven in the evening. But no, she had to wait until I was fully asleep, until the rats and the foxes were out. All this premeditated shit just makes it worse, just makes me think she's out to drive me completely insane.

She makes me want to OD again, for real this time. She makes me want to drink an entire bottle of vodka, even though I can't stand the stuff. She makes me feel like the desperate suicide of women ripped apart by their own insecurity. I have become a monotonous drone and I hate this woman for making me like this. I hate her so much it hurts, it hurts so much that the crazy little thoughts come flooding back into my memory. Thoughts of my killing her, smothering her to death with something. Or something more brutal, like skewering her with a medieval spear (though I don't know where I'd get the spear). These thoughts of murder keep me from completely tipping over, and breaking down into gelatine.

Because I think of life as a series of events, I can place Stella as one of these events. She is an event that I must endure in order to move on to the next and the next and the next. But she is like spiders or snakes, and although I know my life depends on just making it past this pit, I am too repulsed by her to endure anymore.

I wish I could find respite in promiscuity, in the meaningless one-night-stands of self-proclaimed whores, or those with Borderline Personality Disorder.

The drugs are not enough. They don't last long enough to fully block her out. I need something else to prolong the emptiness that comes with being so incredibly stoned. That or 'Eternal Sunshine of the Spotless Mind,' shock therapy, or a series of drugs that would eradicate chosen memories from my temporal lobe. I feel if I have to look at her one more time I may die of overexposure. Overexposure to what though? – I don't even know what she is.

I slowly come to realise that I feel sorry for myself. I don't want to, self-pity is not an attractive quality in a person and I try to be positive, to inject some tone into my monotonous drawl. But somewhere amid all this worrying and self-doubt, I am suckered in by the pathos that surrounds my life like a halo. Ironically evil, as if taking the piss out of everything that a halo should stand for.

I dream that she is beating me up in my sleep, and when I wake my body is bruised and torn and my muscles ache. These episodes leave me in constant pain and a state of perpetual lethargy.

It's after one of these episodes that I realise something has to give, something has got to happen, to change, in order to pull us out of this. So I try being civil, try not to leave a room whenever she enters it. But it's too hard, or it

DRIPFEED

won't work. No matter what I do she's always there to criticise me.

What gets me most, aside from all the jibes and digs at me are the falseness and the split personality bullshit. It's all the fucking hypocrisy and double standardness she exudes; one rule for me, and another for her and Alice. It's okay for Alice to get in trouble at school, but when I did it I got the shit kicked out of me. And herein lies my biggest problem, when I was bad I was bad. When I stayed out all night stoned up to my eyeballs on wacky backy, there was legitimate cause for all the nit picking and arse-kicking and so forth and so forth. But now, now that I've got my shit together, have my A grades and my place in uni, she's treating me like some kind of screw-up. Perhaps in her backwards world she is actually jealous of my success, of my progress from being just another teen delinquent to this.

Weren't we all left with the same deep, penetrating scar tissue that left us incapable of loving? Weren't we all damned from conception – or was that just me? Was I the only one destined to stray from that path of moral righteousness, to be the social fuck-up, the one parents wanted as far away from their little angels as the laws of physics allow? I should have ended up in jail, or out under a bridge somewhere, wrapped in layers in the middle of summer, inside a cardboard box. She expected me to fail, and now that I haven't, she's disappointed because I proved her wrong.

I marvel at how well she can deceive the outside world into believing she is mother of the year. How she can turn on the tears at my bedside and clutch my hand while I'm having my stomach pumped. How she can even claw at the cupboard door while I'm inside slicing the hell out of my wrists. She does these things for the benefit of an audience, any audience, so no one can turn around and get at my real problem, get why I'm really so damaged beyond repair. Stella destroyed me.

I think what I'm missing amid this obvious breakdown is a rock. I read *Prozac Nation,* and note how down and out Elizabeth Wurtzel was feeling. How she couldn't get out of bed for days and the slightest push triggered one of her 'manic' episodes. And I try to determine the differences between us. What it was they set us so far apart, aside of course, from the fact that she was an Ivy League genius and I am barely passing my A levels. But what it all boils down to, once again, is Stella. Wurtzel always had her mother there, to grab her by the lapels and tell her to snap out of it or else. As annoying as it may have seemed, it worked. She got the therapists and the Prozac, the lithium and the love. I got nothing. I am completely alone in this world and it depresses the hell out of me. I am not, however, depressed, which is where Ms. Wurtzel appears to have the upper hand. I am not depressed so psychotropic drugs won't make my demons go away. I can't be cured by therapy and talk. My problem is physical, it is living and breathing, and the minute I am away from it I'll be fine.

DRIPFEED

Keep telling yourself that, says my conscience.
"Fuck off!" I say in response.

I decide to make a conscious effort to kick the dirty habit. Ezra and I decide to quit the junk together. We will be our own sponsors, our own AA meetings, we will do this and we will see it through to the end. Of course real life doesn't work like in the movies, and after a week of self-detox, we are back under Ezra's duvet sharing needles and watching Jeremy Kyle on ITV. I welcome this relapse as a chance to get away from Stella and Alice and their Partridge Family veneer.

Chavez is here too, under the duvet with us, eating KFC because we all get the munchies when we've been smoking that green. "Want me to shoot you up Puss?" Chavez asks, holding the syringe in one hand and the chicken in the other. I'm too strung out to resist temptation, or to even make use of my vocal chords. I offer out my limp arm and smile as she attaches the belt, locates the vein and plunges the needle into its green depths, drawing blood then administering the drug.

Having not done heroin for almost two weeks, I get the exhilarating rush of a first time user. It's better than sex (at least any sex I've ever had, which wasn't good at all). I feel like I could do anything, be anything - so when Chavez leans over and kisses me, I relax and let it happen.

Later on, at uni, I will use this first kiss as a means of getting respect. I will be known as the girl who really has done everything. But for now, with the belt still attached to my arm, and the needle collecting dust on the floor, I kick back in my euphoric, heroin-induced state, and allow Chavez to seduce me.

"Get a fucking room!" Ezra yells, before laughing at the irony and doing a line of coke. "We are so waste," he continues. "Bare fucking waste youths innit." - His south-east London ghetto-boy stylie.

While Chavez gets to work exploring my neck I wonder why Ezra's parents never catch us using his room as our twisted little crack den. On the days when we're ill, when we're lying under the duvet popping Lockets like Fruit Pastels, they're in here, with chicken soup and endless blue packets of Kleenex. Or when we're fine and we're just bumming around sober as fuck and they're still in here, taking pictures of us and contributing towards our debates over the pros and cons of communism and capitalism.

Ezra has the retro kind of avant-garde, hippy type parents we all wish we had. They were the ones who rode around in a hippy wagon in the seventies (ten years too late). They flounce around in tie-dyed shirts and bare feet. They gave Ezra his first spliff.

I compare Ezra's parents to mine. His über-cool nuclear family against my pyscho bitch mother, non-existent father and sociopathic little sister. In the tug of war over who has the best family, mine lose hands down. I wish they were here now, Ezra's parents, they would know how much coke was too much – although class A's aren't really their thing, they draw the line at ecstasy.

Chavez detaches herself from my neck long enough to empty a bag of coke onto an already dusty mirror and sort it into even white lines. Ezra is totally fucked, even I can see that, one more hit of this stuff will send him over the edge, tell his parents that ecstasy is just the doorway to the world we've been experiencing; we live for class A's, if anything at all.

"This is some good shit!" Chavez exclaims as she comes up from the mirror gasping. She wipes her streaming eyes and passes the mirror to me.

I know my limits, and I know that I have already exceeded them. I've already crossed that red line set out to protect teenage crack heads like us from accidental overdose. I've already had two hits of smack, a spliff and a couple of lines of coke, yet I'm about to do two more. This is me all over, the idiot who knows what they're doing is wrong but still makes a conscious effort to go ahead and do it anyway. I take the mirror and the money and sniff that shit, right up my nasal passage. It strikes my brain like tiny pricks of pepper, and I fall back against Chavez, who catches me and prevents me from falling any further.

Later, when we are stoned enough to still be stoned, but sober enough to function, we have the random conversations of those who have done too much coke, and I marvel at how I'm still here, instead of in an emergency room somewhere foaming at the mouth and gasping for air. It hits me here, that maybe Stella hates me because I am a screw-up. Maybe A grades and a place in university aren't enough. Maybe she wants me T-total as well.

I laugh out loud. "What?" both Ezra and Chavez slur at the same time.

"We're so fucking retarded," I say. "We're sitting here smashed out of our heads when we should be out there experiencing."

"Experiencing what Puss?" Chavez asks.

"London!"

"What for?" Ezra asks, suddenly very sober. "When you've lived in London all your life how can you still be excited by it? It's all the same, the same museums and theatres we've been seeing constantly throughout primary school. Or Bond Street and the London Underground. Fuck "experiencing," there's nothing left to experience. How is this shit even exciting anymore?"

He's right, London isn't exciting, not when you've lived in it all your life, seen the same sky and the same trees. The same cars coming out every year under different names. It's not innovative and new anymore; it's dull and boring. I don't even know what I meant when I said that. The

DRIPFEED

only people who can honestly agree with their 'I heart Lndn' t-shirts, are the people experiencing it for the first time. When you've actually lived it, you start to see the rain and the muggings and the cat shit on your lawn.

"Do you think we're addicted?" I ask into the air.
"Of course we are," says Chavez. "Everyone in London's addicted to something baby."

"Yeah –" I am suddenly engulfed by a cold wave of panic. "But are we *dying*?" Chavez closes her eyes, blocking me out, and lights a cigarette, using my neon pink lighter. She offers me the cigarette but I refuse. I'm not interested. I'm not interested in anything anymore, except the random questions no one can be bothered to answer.

I like these times at Ezra's house. For one, we don't do my house anymore, not since Stella went all schizoid and started waking me up at two in the morning to clean her house. Plus, Ezra has a queen-sized bed and an endless supply of junk to get high with. At Ezra's I can get away from Alice's Argos clippings and Stella's bullshit. I can even get away from myself for a while. When I'm around here, with Ezra and Chavez, the voices in my head stop telling me I'm worthless and instead sing my praises, telling me I am an invincible thing of beauty.

This house is like a rainbow, or *Buttermoon*. It is bathed in the elixir of eternal happiness, and it brings me such joy just to bask in its sunshine. This is the complete opposite to my house, my Addams Family dungeon. My house is like a black hole that drains my happiness. Once I'm in there, it seems like I even forget how to smile. Once inside that place, a smile looks weird on me, like I'm faking it or grimacing in pain.

Back in my dungeon I go straight to my room, which is the only place I'm allowed to go since Stella started locking doors to keep me out, or herself in. I drop my keys on the table and pick up my phone, which I forgot to bring with me today. I have four missed calls – all from Belle – and a voicemail. T-mobile is being a bitch and charging its customers to retrieve voicemails, and since I have no credit, this will go unlistened to.

I don't know what to do here, except watch terrestrial television and fall asleep. I contemplate slitting my wrists again, just so I'll have something to do, but I'm not in that dark place anymore and I'd be too scared to press the knife down properly. In my lack of things to do, I call Belle from my house phone; not even caring that I'm not allowed to use it and when Stella finds out she'll probably behead me. It's already after one, but Belle agrees to meet me on Tottenham Court road where a new club is set to open. Neither of us remembers what it's called, but it's exclusive; brand new, beds and shit. Plus, it's only five pounds to get in and the music will be so loud I won't have to listen to Belle's bullshit.

DRIPFEED

I don't have a car and since it's after the last train, I have to call for a cab. The cab only costs me twenty pounds, which is twenty pounds more than I can afford, but I also can't afford to spend yet another night at home staring at the walls waiting for Stella's sleeping pills to wear off. She'll get pissed off and make me perform some menial task or other. At least this way she won't even know I'm gone.

The cab ride from my house through middle-classed suburbia makes me feel guilty. Whenever I'm away from Stella for too long, I start to forget what she's really like and I start feeling guilty about taking advantage, or the piss, whatever. In the cab, riding through the suburbs where all the lights are off and all the cars are parked in their respective drives, I start to feel that maybe this is not a good idea; maybe *I* should be at home, in my dark house, sleeping like the rest of these kids.

Though I am feeling incredibly guilty, it doesn't once occur to me to just turn around and go home. I sit here, in the back seat, fantasising about what may or may not lay ahead of me.

We get to the club, which is heaving considering it's only two and the club doesn't close for another six hours. Belle is outside looking haughty and condescending as usual. Midnight nails and blood red lips, she looks like she just stepped out of *Nosferatu*. We go in and I spot the lead singer from indie/rock band *Basement* standing by one of the beds holding a bottle of Grolsch, swaying to the music and looking all smouldering. Belle winks at him and gives me a pinch on the arm, like we're girlfriends or something, not bothering, or not caring, that we are both only here due to lack of other alternative.

Somehow, I don't know, we – Belle and I – end up in some scummy little back room that smells like piss and arse, with the lead singer from *Basement,* whose name I can't be bothered to find out. Belle and lead singer sit on empty milk crates doing lines and swapping battle scars; tales of promiscuous one nighters, bouts with the black cloud and near death experiences. I feel like jumping in and saying, "You want some real dirt? Wanna hear about the time I OD'd? And that shit was not accidental." But I don't say any of this, I just sit there on my own milk crate, listening to the two of them laughing and joking, feeling more and more like a third wheel.

Eventually, it seems like so much time has passed since we got here, another member of *Basement*, the drummer Howie, shows up with a fresh bag of coke and enough charm to distract me from this evening. Just as the night is starting to seem less shit, Belle turns to me and reminds me why I hate her so much. "Yo Chuck," she calls. "I didn't know you were in to guys! Where's your girlfriend?"

Howie turns and looks at me like he just won the jackpot. "Girlfriend," he repeats.

"Yeah," I say snatching the bag from him and sorting it on the floor. "I'm just a big, fat, scary dyke." Howie seems to think this is the funniest

DRIPFEED

thing he has ever heard. What I find funny at this point is how desperation can cause people to do stupid things, and the lengths some people - namely me - will go to, just to get that first high they've been searching forever to find. Here I am, on my hands and knees, snorting coke off the floor while some stranger tells me how hot it would be to fuck me and my girlfriend. I don't even bother telling him that Chavez is *not* my girlfriend, that I'm not even gay, that the only thing I want to do right now is get these lines off the floor and into my nose. When I come up for air, I realise that Belle has disappeared off somewhere with lead-singer-guy. Unlike me, Belle is able to engage in meaningless, casual sex with random guys in skinny jeans and pointy boots; she's probably outside right now screwing the brains out of the lead singer.

The music from the other room seems muffled and far away. The amount of drugs I've done today has practically fried my brain and Howie is actually starting to look quite sexy, the way he's staring at me with those dark, bedroom eyes.
Maybe I've got this Borderline Personality Disorder thing like Susanna Kaysen, embarking upon one meaningless sex act after another. Maybe I am crazy after all, except I didn't sleep with Chavez and I haven't even kissed Howie yet. Not to worry though, two more hits and I'll be there.

After my sixth line of the evening, Howie and I locate Belle and lead singer, whose name is Stewie. I can't help thinking that Howie and Stewie sounds like some sort of gimmick, like if I'd known about this before I could never have taken this band seriously. We jump into some beat-up old cars, which appear around the corner, and head back to theirs. Inside the flat Stewie and Belle disappear; leaving Howie and I to our own devices, to do whatever it is we came here to do.

"So your girlfriend..." he almost asks.

"What about her?" I say whilst licking the sticky side of a rizla.

"No worries," he says. I don't know, or care, what this means. Instead I light the spliff with the neon pink lighter and inhale, wondering how much more shit I'll have to take tonight before I OD again.

"So?" says Howie, taking the spliff from me, inhaling and blowing smoke rings out at me.

"What?" I ask. "And how do you blow smoke rings like that? I've never been able to do that." I love the way that, even though he's probably done as much shit as I have tonight – if not more, Howie still looks sober enough to drive. His pupils aren't even dilated, and while my eyes are clearly bloodshot, his are perfectly white.

"So," he repeats. A statement this time, not a question. I take the spliff back from him and make the mistake of standing up, getting both the cocaine and head rush at the same time. My heart is beating so fast it feels like Michael Flatly is tap-dancing in there. I get the sudden urge to go

DRIPFEED

and drink water. Instead of going to the kitchen tap like any normal person, I end up in the bathroom, experiencing my euphoric cocaine high twelve hits too late and collapsing in the bathtub. Drummer guy (I've forgotten his name again) joins me presently.

We fuck, screw, knock boots, whatever.

I'm not sure I'll remember this in the morning. It's already seven.

I wake up, still naked, still in the bathtub, and still stoned, at ten thirty later on that morning. Judging by the state of me, and of Howie, I got my wish to be promiscuous and engage in that meaningless one-night-stand I wanted. Except this is not what I expected. Even though I'm still stoned, I'm sober enough to remember every single detail of last nights little shenanigans, and I am deeply ashamed. Here I am, naked and stoned in a bathtub, having spent the last few hours screwing the brains of some man I just met on a milk crate, and instead of feeling new and liberated like I was supposed to, I feel like a cheap tacky Christmas decoration. I have become the cliché of the fucked-up teenager and the rock star – except Howie is hardly a rock star, and I'm hardly that fucked-up.

The worst thing about last night was not the drugs, or the sex. The worst thing, for me, was the aftermath that manifests itself through these feelings of worthlessness and self-pity. I am so disgusted with myself that I don't even want to look in the mirror as I walk past it, trying to leave the flat without waking anyone up. I'm not even thinking of what Stella will say when I stroll in through the door; she'll probably wave a drunken hand in my face and rip me apart when she's good and sober.

I manage to disentangle myself from Howie without waking him up. I manage to get my clothes on and get out of the door without waking anyone up. Once I'm out of the door though, I realise how much of a loss I'm really at. Since we drove here, at night, I have no idea where I am, and how to get home. I end up walking miles to the train station, before realising that I don't even have enough money for a travel card. I go to call Ezra, hoping he'll be able to arrange a lift for me. Then I realise I left my phone at home again, and even if I had it, I don't have credit on it, so it's pretty much useless anyway.

    I manage to persuade the man protecting the barriers of East Finchley train station that I'm stranded. He must see my desperation, because he issues me with a temporary pass, the kind they give you when you've been caught bunking, and he sends me on my way.

By the time I get home, I'm too tired and weak to listen to Alice talk about how many kinds of atom there are, or exactly how long it's going to take for the sun to shrivel up and die. I kick her out of the way, side-stepping the pieces of cut-up paper

DRIPFEED

she's placed on the floor to keep me boxed in, and go up to my room.

"Why don't you like me?" she yells from the bottom of the stairs. I fall onto my unmade bed that is still messy from yesterday, and fall asleep fully clothed. At some point the phone rings, but it isn't in my room, and to get up in my present state would be way too painful. I lay on the bed asleep but awake, while the ringing phone slices through my brain. Perhaps the phone is ringing in my head. Perhaps it isn't ringing at all.

It seems as if this little act of mine finally gave me the balls I needed to kick back at Stella and tell her what I really think.

"Where were you last night?" she screams after bursting into my room.

"What do you care?" I say in my usual monotonous drawl.

"Why do you do this? What is wrong with you? Do you want to shame me? Is that it? Do you want to lay me bare and naked on the front lawn for all the neighbours to see? Is that what you want, Charlotte?"

"Oh for fucks sake, Stella," I say, finally snapping. "Me, me, me. It's always about you. Just because you're husbandless and friendless, no job, no degree, no prospects, don't take your shortcomings out on me. I didn't ask you to run away and have kids; I didn't even ask to be born. If you wanted a silent, stress-free life, maybe you should have joined a convent, or run away to a mountain somewhere."

"Charlotte."

"Don't, fucking call me that, *Stella!*" I am screaming at her now. "I keep telling you that Charlotte's not here, and you keep acting like I am. My. Name. Is. Chuck!"

Silence.

Stella is crying now, not huge, gulping, attention-seeking tears like I do, but real, silent tears of complete and utter defeat. And I don't care that she's crying. I am finally feeling the indifference I wanted so badly to feel. These could be the last tears of a dying worm for all I care.

"Ah, that's bare rude," Ezra says when I tell him about Howie and Stella, and me making the latter cry.

"No, it's not, she deserved it." I don't tell Ezra that Howie has already called three times since that night, that I've purposefully missed the call each time. This was meant to be a meaningless one-nighter, not the beginnings of a new relationship.

Maybe it's true; maybe whoever said women were eternally dissatisfied was right. Or maybe it's just humanity in general. In winter we long for summer, but when it finally gets here we complain about the heat and beg for a chill, which, when it finally arrives again, we are completely upset by. I wanted a one-nighter, which I got – perhaps I even wanted a relationship out of it, secretly though, and now that it's here, now that it's right in front of my face, I don't want it anymore. It's not that I'm of the 'love-em-and-leave-em' variety; I just can't be arsed.

"But she's your mum," Ezra continues, not understanding that not everyone has parents like his.

"Not everyone has perfect parents like yours you know," I tell him. "Shit!"

It's funny how we always want what we can't have but then when we actually get it we don't want it anymore. We are spared the fruits of our own labour purely because we can't make our fucking minds up. Howie was the perfect example of that: couldn't have him, wanted him, got him, didn't want him. Humans aren't all that complex, in fact, we are really, really, outstandingly simple. We're so predictable it's almost laughable. We're like the mice in the cage that keep going for the cheese even though they know it will shock them. Not only are we predictable and boring, we are also stupid as well. We keep running into the same brick wall time and time again, because we are too stupid to register the pain. "Cause and effect," can't even be used here. It's just effect, effect, effect. We effectively destroy ourselves, and the worst thing is we are so predictable we even see it coming; we don't even try to get out of the way before it hits.

We live life like we're in a movie, always expecting that miracle, waiting for the good things to come and take us away from those melancholic routines. But real life is a routine; we get up, we brush our teeth, we go to work. Then we come home, brush our teeth, take a shit, and go to bed. No helicopters, no axe-murderers, no talking, homicidal dolls, just plain old predictable human beings and their Monday mornings and casual Fridays.

The trouble is we need all that Hollywood shit to even out the balance. Take it away and all we're left with is our own morbid humanity, the feeling that, any day now, we're all going to keel over and die, one by one. It's because of thoughts like this that my friends are growing tired of me. Because I say things like, 'my feet are bouncy', or, 'maybe it was the aliens,' people don't know how to receive me. Why bother? I think. Why not just leave me unreceived, unclaimed in the lost-and-found of a Megabus depot. Who even cares anymore? I am random and profound and that suits me just fine. My profundity is tailored to my size eight-ness, who cares if no one else gets it?

I think of getting a tattoo, getting some deep, profound, Latin phrase branded upon my skin. Like *quod natura non sunt turpia* – so people can fully understand my desire to be detached. I am my own inspiration, and I aspire to be me. This nondescript, uncaring-ness, is often mistaken for arrogance. I am arrogant because I don't care, or because I do care. Either way I can't win. Either way, '*brevoir saltare cum deformibus virus est vita.*' Flies will always fly in through open windows, and my bed sheets will always be stained with the ink from writing too much meaningless bullshit on

DRIPFEED

the crux of finding out who I really am. Everything in Latin sounds profound.

A fly buzzing in my face can make me so nervous, so anxious and agitated, that I can write an entire essay on how overwrought and fucked-up I am, but will be unable to read it later because my fucking hand was shaking so much. This is me now; I break out in hot, prickly sweats at loud noises. This is why lightning scares the shit out of me, and thunder reduces me to a quivering wreck underneath the duvet, lacking in the common sense to just switch the light on.
      Perhaps I have Parkinson's disease, because my hands won't stop shaking and I'm so edgy and highly-strung all the time. How can I be so calm and relaxed one minute, and turn into a paranoid schizo the next? Switching so sporadically between these two polar extremes can't possibly be good for my anxiety. Who knows, maybe the world really is involved in some warped conspiracy theory to slaughter me for being too crazy, or not crazy enough. Whatever. Either way I'm constantly looking over my shoulder, constantly running away from nothing, or from the prospect of nothingness.

Gradually the summer wears on and university seems like more than just an urban myth, it seems like two months away. I avoid seeing Belle altogether, her miasmatic presence is more than I can handle. She is positively noxious, just breathing her in is damaging to my health. I cannot be in any more back rooms, on a milk crate, while she's shedding skin with lead singers of rock bands and breathing, too heavily, in alleyways outside. This reminds me that I still haven't returned any of Howie's calls, not that I want a repeat performance of last night. Not that I even need him, not now.

DRIPFEED

Chapter 4

I spend most of my days bumming around alone – avoiding the home front. I am alone because I renounced Belle, and Ezra has found a job as a stylist for Miss Selfridge. Most of the time I hang out in Starbucks, eating blueberry cheesecake and drinking my money away. The amount of money I've spent in the there I could have probably used to invest in my own line of classy coffee houses.

Much of the time spent in Starbucks is used contemplating, mulling things over and conversing with the voices in my head over what I should do next. Or rather, what I should do *before* what I do next, which is – ultimately – to attend university and gain my respectful place amongst the scholars and lecturers.

One day when I'm in Starbucks, at eleven in the morning, having a deep and meaningless conversation with myself, a woman comes over, with a black coffee, and sits at my table. She looks at me with this really perplexed expression, kind of like the way Chavez looked at me in the beginning, when I knew her as Maria.

"Shouldn't you be at school?" the woman asks.

"Shouldn't you be at work?" I retort. The woman smiles at me.

"Actually, yes," she says.

"Well I guess we're both fucked then, aren't we?" This woman is so obviously hitting on me, which I find quite hilarious. What I find even funnier, is that I don't mind, which makes me think that perhaps Chavez succeeded in transforming me or whatever it is she did.

"Coffee?" the woman asks.

"When in Starbucks…"

She laughs then and says, "You're much too witty to be in school."

The woman turns out to be Diane or Diana – some thirty-something year old corporate tycoon who happens to have a thing for eighteen year old girls. I let her buy me the coffee (and cheesecake); I even let her take me out to lunch and dinner a few times. I even go to her flat, which is in trendy Notting Hill, the playpen of all the young trendy business-types.

Her house is the kind you see on *Grand Designs,* where a couple build a house or convert a flat, and you find yourself hating these strangers because you know you will never own a house quite like it, and even if it is – quite like it – it won't be the same because you just ripped it from the people on *Grand Designs.*

The flat is a converted Victorian house – converted into two flats – and is all quaint and periodic on the outside, but is ultra modern and stream-lined on the in. Hardwood floors, stainless steel kitchen units, and black leather sofas. It does kind of defeat the objective of buying period – not that I care, but there are no original features,

DRIPFEED

bar an antique fireplace, which doesn't even work. The whole flat gives the impression of some public-schooled playboy, playing with daddy's credit cards.

Now that I'm here in the house, I feel like I've crossed another of those imaginary lines I'm so prone to crossing these days. I feel obligated, like I did with Howie, to repay this woman for bringing me here. And I'm not even into women, Chavez was an exception. Diane puts on music (which has got to be an invitation), some sedate jazz that emanates from her ultra-sleek, high-tech stereo system. The music means what I thought has been confirmed, this woman expects more from me than I am prepared to give.

"Do you mind if I use your bathroom?" I ask.

"Of course not, it's down the hall on the right."

Bathrooms are always 'down the hall.' I go in, lock the door, and sit on the toilet seat. I have roughly five minutes to devise my escape plan before Diane/Diana comes looking for me. I could go out the window, though it's hardly big enough and I'd get stuck halfway. I could sneak down the stairs, hoping they're not creaky like mine, or, I could just go down and face the fucking music. I made the choice to accept that cup of coffee and those invitations of dinner, to come here – to swanky Notting hill – even though it's way out of my way. Or I could just go down and tell the truth, explain that I'm just a spineless little girl whose only intention was to prove, to myself, that I can be daring and spontaneous as well as stupid and irrational.

I end up spending so long in the bathroom that Diane has to come upstairs and bang on the door to see if I'm alright. I reach over and open the door, even though I'm still sitting on the toilet. Diane comes in and kneels down in front of me.

"You know you don't have to do this if you don't want to," she says. "I'll take you home, if you want."

Saying 'yes please, take me home now' would seem so childish; Diane would think I was just another waste of her time. But there are no alternatives to this: stay and do something I really don't want to, or go home and watch *Hollyoaks*.

We get into Diane's BMW and she drives me home. I am ashamed and embarrassed, because I led this woman on, gave her false hope and wasted her time. I can't even look at her. I scoot as far away from her as I can in the passengers seat, and keep my eyes on the droplets of rain falling onto the windscreen. It's really funny, how the weather always changes to affect my mood. Like *Romeo and Juliet,* the bit where Mecrucio dies and the weather turns into a storm.

"Don't worry about it," Diane is saying. "Don't look so stressed."

"I'm not stressed," I grumble. I am fully aware that I now sound like a spoilt teenager.

"What's wrong then?" She keeps her eyes on the road, and I get the impression that she's fed up with me too; just like everyone else is – and she's only known me a week, I really know how to turn people off.

"I'm sad," I say mechanically.

"Why are you sad?"

"Because living at home has become so unbearable I'd rather die than spend another minute there. Because I don't think I can make it through the next ten weeks. Because even though I really, really don't want to die, I keep getting these urges to kill myself and they're getting stronger and stronger every day. Because right now, I'm desperate for any other alternative to this." She actually stops the car here, because she is one of the people for whom the phrases *big heart* and *sucker for a sob story* are meant. She turns and looks at me, and in the instance between our eyes locking and me looking away – because I think she's hitting on me again – I see something I have never seen before. This woman barely knows me, yet she looked at me like she really gave a shit.

"Have you told anyone this?" she asks.

"You mean besides you?"

"Yes."

I laugh, loud, raucous, hysterical laughter; the kind that warrants sedation. I'm laughing so hard that the car is actually shaking and Diane is looking at me with something between fear and amusement. This is funny, this is more than funny, this is positively hilarious. The very thought of telling anyone what I just told this stranger has never once crossed my mind. They would look at me like I was some kind of nutcase, which I probably am. I could never divulge such top secret information.

"Now I'm worried, Chuck," she says quietly, like she's my shrink and I just detailed ten ways I'd like to kill myself. And I'm still laughing, because this is funny shit; laughter is infectious, it spreads like disease and becomes uncontrollable. "I'm worried," she repeats again. And the laughter stops suddenly, like it started, and I'm me again.

"Don't be," I say. "I'm fine. Just carry on driving." Diane doesn't start driving again. She stares out at the rain as if I'm her problem. "You must think I'm crazy," I say, to fill the silent chasm. "I hear voices in my head as well, just in case you were wondering." The laughter starts again, more suddenly this time.

"I don't think you're crazy. I think you need help"

DON'T SAY IT!
"I think..."
SHIT!
"I think..."
HERE IT COMES!
"I think you're depressed."
!!!!!!!!!!!!!!!!!!!!!!!!!

Aww man, she had to go and use the 'D' word; had to go assuming I'm depressed 'cause I said I had urges to kill myself. What's the deal with that? I said I didn't want to die didn't I? Women are too perceptive by far, reading into things that really aren't there. I can't help stressing to myself, that I do not know this woman, yet here she is, psychoanalysing me, preparing to

DRIPFEED

have me carted off to a day-care centre where they'll stick a thermometer in my mouth and make it better.

Diane refuses to move the car until I promise not to do anything stupid; to stay away from sharp objects and tiny white sleeping pills. Only when I convince her that she has, by diagnosing my problem, effectively saved me from myself and eradicated my suicidal tendencies, does she continue to drive towards the suburbs. Though she keeps looking at me from the corner of her eye, probably scared I've got a .22 hidden up my sleeve, or worse, a packet of pills and a bottle of Vodka.

I make her drop me off at the top of my road; it wouldn't do to have Stella see me stepping out of the BMW; she'd be over there demanding to know what man I've been fucking for money - oh what little faith in me she has, and what little she really knows.

When I get through the doors the house is buzzing with people and children hanging around eating sausages off cocktail sticks, and drinking glasses of wine or bottles of J20. It is a surprise I didn't hear the noise from outside the door.

Stella has her mask on today, the plastic veneer she uses to disguise what this house really is. Even Alice is here, not quoting Anton LeVay or trailing pieces of glue and magazine all over the place. She looks like any other normal kid in faded Levis and pink bows. Something about this scene is wrong, the way

Stella doesn't rush to drag me over to her side where she sings my praises to her "friends" and showers me with champagne. The way she doesn't even acknowledge my existence is quite unnerving in itself. I want her to stop and tell me *she's* worried about me, not some dyke-bitch stranger in a BMW. I want *Stella* to stop me from damaging myself any further. She's given up on me now, or she just doesn't want the burden of me anymore.

"Why didn't you come down?" Stella asks the next morning, forgetting all about the fact that she – on two separate occasions – woke me up in the ungodly hours of the morning to clean dust off pennies. "Everyone was there," she continues. "You should have come down." She looks at me with that perplexed expression everyone seems to be adopting with me these days.

"Why?" I ask, genuinely wanting to know why this woman would want me anywhere near her at a time when she is obviously in entertainment mode, at a time where she obviously has so much to lose. Somehow, because she's sober and because she's being nice to me, I forget how much of a bitch she can be, and I actually mistake this lapse in real character for genuine concern. I actually start feeling bad for my indifference, and my failure to attend her impromptu cocktail party.

Stella doesn't even bother to answer the question. She could have gone for something cheesy like, 'because you're my daughter and I love you,' even though I would have seen right through that, the effort would have been nice. The fact that she says nothing, just stares at me with eyes that are slowly becoming hazy and unfocused, confirms all my previous suspicions. Funnily enough, there is no audience here in my bedroom, and I can only assume this little performance is for my benefit. Doesn't she know that I know? How dare she pretend to me?

Stella switches back to normal as the pills or alcohol kick in. "Your room is filthy," she says. "You should clean it."

I wish I had the kind of mother who sat on the edge of my bed braiding my hair and teasing me about the boy I fancied who, although didn't fancy me back, was thoroughly overjoyed by the idea of me as his lap dog. The kind who gave advice that I would sneer at to her face but secretly take later on. We got on well back in the day, back when I was her little Cheerio and she took me to work with her, where she cleaned other people's floors with formaldehyde in plastic buckets. She braided my hair *then*, painted my toenails and made videos of me singing along to the soundtrack of *Grease*. I never could have imagined those days would ever end; now, I can't believe they ever existed. I have become the kind of person she detests; the eccentric, arrogant kind who doesn't give a fuck about what the person behind her is saying about her.

Perhaps I should have made more of an effort to be her friend; she did – after all – give up her life and education to raise me. She gave up the dream of a young twenty-something year old Londoner to wipe shit off my arse and mashed banana off my chin.

Today is a good day, and one of the rare days that I feel almost completely happy. I meet Ezra from Miss Selfridge and we go for a sushi lunch in Prêt. We talk about normal things that normal people can understand, not our usual cryptic riddle-talk. Today we are not stoned, we are completely straight and acting as the perfect pillars of society our parents wanted us to be.

"What's going on with you and Hewie?" Ezra asks.

"Howie," I correct absently. "I dunno, he keeps calling but I can't be bothered to answer. I dunno what to say,"

"Hello?" offers Ezra.

"Funny," I say. "But seriously, it was meant to be a one time thing, and it's been so long. Why is he still calling me?" Ezra gazes out of the window at a couple of Emo boys eating from MacDonald's bags.

"What about that woman then?" He says.

"What about her? I told her I wanted to kill myself and she got all worried and was like, 'I'm not driving until you promise you're okay,' blah, blah, blah. Besides, that's not even what I'm into." Ezra raised an eyebrow, and I know he's thinking about Chavez; the very fact that I'm thinking about Chavez suggests that it *is* what I'm into, and maybe Diane was just too old, or way out of my

DRIPFEED

league. Whatever it was, it was too weird; an older woman and me. It just didn't make sense.

"Wanna fuck shit up at mine later?" Ezra asks.

"Don't you ever think we need to sort it out?" I say slowly. "I mean, all we ever do is 'fuck shit up.' We started out having fun, now we're just a couple of junky bums – or I am, at least you have a job.

Ezra thinks for a minute, "Yeah," he says. "But we're not bums; we're just having fun innit?"

I sigh exasperatedly. "That's what I mean, we're having *too much* fun; it's not even the fun normal people our age are having. It's self-destructive."

"Just cos you sniff aerosols when you run out of coke and slit your wrists every time you get pissed off at your mum."

"I'm allowed to do that," I reply. "I'm fucked-up innit."

"We're all fucked-up." We've finish our sushi and prepare to leave Prêt; Ezra still has ages left on his lunch break so we head down to Topshop to check out the sales. "So," inquires Ezra. "Are we gonna fuck shit up or not? I can call Charlie and Chavez – I know you don't like Belle." This is my problem. This is why I'm so fucked-up; because I make grandeur fucking speeches, where I rip apart some stupid aspect of my life, and then, right after I've done it, I go right ahead and contradict myself by taking part or saying 'yes.' And there I was complaining about

Stella's hypocrisy, not bothering to take note of my own.

"Yeah," I say. "And for the record, I don't like Charlie either. He fancies you, you know."

"Cos I'm bare buff innit," Ezra says. "What do you think of these?" He holds up a pair of grey Moto skinny jeans that have been reduced to five pounds in the sale.

"For you or for me?" I ask.

"Me of course."

"Go for it," I say, even though I don't understand why gay boys feel the need to wear women's clothing, I mean, there's a Topman right up the escalator, where I'm sure he'd find a pair of perfectly skinny man-jeans.

"Give me your NUS!" Ezra demands. We are lucky enough to look alike and I hand it over.

"Wait a minute!" I say. "Basement are playing Underworld tonight, I saw a flyer in Howie's flat. D'you wanna go there instead?"

"Do they search at the door?"

"Come on, Ezra, it's Camden not Leicester Square."

We leave Topshop, Ezra with his one pair of jeans, me with my nothing, and I walk Ezra up Great Portland Street and back to work. I briefly think about checking Carnaby Street out, since I want to get this new pair of Vans, but now that Ezra's gone and I'm all alone I'm feeling really down again. All I want to do is curl up on the floor in my bedroom and do a couple of lines, and if I haven't got anymore coke, maybe I will do some

DRIPFEED

aerosols. Ezra was wrong, I don't sniff glue and all that shit, I heard about a kid doing it once and then dying; but now, now that Ezra's planted the seed, I feel I owe it to myself to at least try it out.

I head down to Oxford Street tube station – which is surprisingly packed and sweaty considering it's only three in the afternoon – and who should I bump in to but Howie, *Basement*.

"Chuck! Right?" he asks, like he hasn't been plaguing my phone with texts and voicemails for the past couple of weeks.

"Howie!" I exclaim, finding it hard to believe that I, junky teenage delinquent, could have been so good in bed – drunk and all – that this grown, twenty-something year old man, could be so plagued by the mere absence of me he feels the need to stalk me via T-mobile. I know, without asking, that whatever line I get will 'just happen' to be his line, and that wherever I go, he'll be going too. I'll be forced to engage in fruitless conversation for the twenty minutes it takes to get to Victoria, the fifteen minutes it then takes to get to Charring Cross, and then, if he dares, the twenty minutes it takes to get back home to middle-classed suburbia.

He doesn't bother asking what was wrong with my phone, or why I haven't replied to his texts or voicemails, and I don't bother asking how he even got my number in the first place – I know Belle thought she was doing me a great disservice by handing it over the morning after I left.

"Are you coming tonight?" he asks.

I don't want to sound desperate and too eager, like he does. "Maybe," I say. "If I can find some money."

"I'll put you on guest list if you want?"

What is it about men? One minute they're claiming how, even though they'd gladly fuck a one-night-stand, they'd have no respect for her the next morning. Here I am, or there I was, engaging in the very act that should have labelled me *whore* or *slut*, and here he is hanging onto my ankles, preventing me from moving anywhere.

"You don't have to," I say.

"Nah, s'cool, we get too many places anyway. And if you don't have any money…"

"Yeah, thanks." So now I have to go. Now I'm obligated, to attend this gig, to spend yet more listless hours naked in a bathtub. Somehow, Howie and I find stuff to talk about: his band, the fact that I've never graced the strings of a guitar or the skin of a drum with anything more than a fingertip. And even though I've only met this man on one other occasion, I find myself drawn to him.

We meet outside the venue as always, Ezra, Charlie, Chavez and I. Even though I hate her, Belle's absence feels strange. Even though I'd rather not have her complaining about my hair or my clothes, or my taste in men, it somehow doesn't feel complete without her here to bitch and moan about whatever pissed her off that day.

There are no swish leather sofas at Underworld; the only seating comes in the form of crusty old

DRIPFEED

wooden benches off in a corner, under some stairs, that smells like shit and arse. Hardly anyone shows up for the first band – a group of seventeen year old boys from South East London – and I wonder just how bad *Basement* are. It isn't until floods of people arrive from nowhere, crushing me where I'm standing, that I realise they actually do have a following of largely depressed indie-kids.

Howie comes out, shirtless, and I see someone wrote a *C* in the middle of his chest; this is ridiculous. Chavez shoots me a look, putting two and two together: the guest list, big *C* on drummer's chest, all this is not a coincidence. She shrugs though, she couldn't care less.

The set lasts half an hour, at the end of which Chavez and I are free to sneak off to the toilets to spike our drinks with rum, and do a quick few lines off a mirror on the seat of a toilet. When we get back out, ever so slightly stoned, Ezra and Charlie are engaged in a deep conversation with Howie – who appears to be waiting for me.

"Nice boyfriend," Charlie whispers to me.

"Fuck off Dildo," I say back.

"Did you like it?" Howie asks me.

"The gig?" I ask back, lighting a Marlboro with my neon pink lighter, and sipping from my spiked drink.

"Yeah, the gig," Howie replies, smiling at the double entendre.

"It was okay."

Lami Okrekson

We end up at Howie's flat again: Ezra and Chavez shooting each other up with Stewie's needles, Charlie smoking green because he doesn't like to share needles, Howie and I sharing a joint in the kitchen – this time I will not get so fucked that I end up naked in the bath!

Now that I'm experiencing this flat semi-sober, I can't help comparing it to Diane's chic, Notting hill abode. The flat itself is impressive for a band of broke twenty-something year old men. It's as nice as any flat in East Finchley can be. The walls are littered with signed posters of bands I have never heard of – and some that I have. This flat seems entirely different to the flat I passed out in three weeks ago. I never noticed all the guitar cases, guitars stacked in racks along the walls, drum sticks all over the floor, and drum kit by the window. How could I have missed all this before? – even the dog bowl on the floor in the kitchen, though there's no dog in sight; perhaps they ate it in times of desperate hunger.

I get back home at four in the morning, having missed the last trains and being forced to night bus it back to my end. This time the house is dark and silent. The usual smells of vodka and Pritt Stick greet me as I open the door, coupled with the faint aromas from the party last night: too much perfume and cologne, sausages, and spilt tomato sauce.

    Back in my room all memories of the last few hours are instantly erased. Alone, I can

DRIPFEED

hardly believe I have friends, least of all the ones who hang out, chillaxing, taking hits on bongs made from empty coke bottles. I can hardly believe I ever had fun. Once again, this house drains my happiness and leaves me feeling desperate and suicidal. While I was hardly having a blast at Howie's, I was at least enjoying myself. Why do I feel so shit now?

The next morning I have absolutely nothing to do. It's a Saturday so Alice is at home, on the stairs reading James Joyce's *Ulesyss* and chewing the ends of her frayed sweater.
"Why do you cut things out of magazines?" I ask her.
"Because they're things I'll need." I don't ask her what she'll ever need a photograph of a meat cleaver for; I just let her get on with the book she's way too young to be reading. I started *Ulesyss* a couple of months ago and didn't even make it past the first page. With nothing else to do I go back to my room, lie on my bed, light a cigarette, and pick up the phone to call Howie.
"Hi it's me," I say; even though his phone has caller ID and *me* could be anyone, if it doesn't.
"Hi," he says back. We go back and forth like this, monosyllabic answers, not really having fun, but also denying each other the right to put the phone down. There are frequent lapses in the conversation, although these are not comfortable silences, they don't phase me. It's not like Ezra, with whom there is never a dull moment over the phone, or Chavez, with whom silences are

comfortable and familiar; Howie and I just don't have that much to say to each other. I've never been much of a talker and I'm hardly one of those girls who can switch on the bubbly happiness whenever. Although I am not remotely gothic, I already have the antisocial, sociopathic tendencies of a goth.

The phone call with Howie only lasted an hour and I am still at a loss for credible things to do. I ran out of coke a few days ago and I can't be bothered to go out and get some, and besides, I'm also running out of money and all the coke is turning me into a zombie. When I reach over for a can of spray paint and an old t-shirt, I think that maybe I am addicted, if not to the drug itself then to the blankness it brings with it. I already use more than both Ezra and Charlie, more even than Chavez – the epitome of teen junkiness. Inhaling the fumes from the t-shirt, I finally realise what all the hot fuss is about. Everything drifts slowly out of my head, and my brain feels completely numb.

    Raucous, uncontrollable laughter comes up in bubbles from the pit of my stomach to the tip of my brain. Any minute now Stella's going to be up here telling me to shut up; like the time I watched *Drop Dead Fred* for the first time and laughed so hard she heard me all the way from the ground floor. This is different to then, this is not hilarity, this is a hazy, lazy kind of funny that seems to have taken over my whole body. I feel weak and I just want to lean back on my bed, drool starts dripping down my chin but I am too weak to wipe it away, so I leave it there, wait a few moments and then do some more. This time it actually knocks me back against the pillow, where I wait for a while, trying to see past my eyes. Then the door opens and Alice walks in, still carrying the big, ugly book.

"Solvent abuse kills!" At least that's what the posters around college used to say. Solvent abuse is often associated with young males between the ages of eleven and sixteen. Sniffing spray cans, glue, lighter fuel, delivers a strong intoxicating kick followed by mild hallucinations; this is why there is three of Alice staring at me right now and why the wallpaper behind her is moving in weird undulating waves. Because the effects of solvent abuse are short-lived, I am completely straight again by the time Alice gets over to my bed.

"Why were you laughing like that?" She demands.

"Something funny happened."

"What happened?"

"The wallpaper moved." Alice must think I'm taking the piss because she storms out of the room muttering something about never wanting to be a teenager, and I hear her regain her place on the steps. I close my eyes and try to go back to sleep. I am tired and lethargic and all I want to do is lay here in the dark.

The days go on like that. Some days I am too tired to anything but lay in bed smoking cigarettes and watching cartoons.

Too much sleep becomes counter-productive and the body actually finds it a huge effort to drag itself out of bed, which, in turn, results in more and more sleep to compensate for the draining effect it has on the brain. This is where I'm at now, too tired to move myself out of this drugged-up inertia, but too frustrated to just lean back and enjoy it. So, like thousands of other junkies, most of whom are my friends, I lay under the duvet listening to Radiohead through earphones, waiting for this thing to hurry up and pass. I wish Chavez were here to shoot me up and make me feel normal, but she isn't, I am completely alone and screaming inside my head.

That is, until Howie calls.

DRIPFEED

Chapter 5

Howie's calls are becoming a regular occurrence – as are my calls to him, and I find myself spending more and more time at his flat, not even there for the drugs, but for the need of him. We have now, unofficially, become somewhat of an item; at least we now fuck sober, as well as completely and utterly trashed. I find myself at every one of *Basement's* gigs, air kissing the girlfriends of its other members – glad to see that the girlfriend Stewie introduces me to, is not Belle, nor does she even resemble Belle in the slightest. Many of the long summer nights are spent outside in their tiny basement garden doing lines or taking hits on a bong, sometimes doing both and ending up passed out on the garden tiles.

Strangely, my 'relationship' (it still makes me cringe to call it that), is having negative effects on my head. After the last overdose, in the cupboard at home, I felt like weights were being lifted off of me and I was okay again. Even Stella seemed far away, like I had acquired a Stella-proof vest to protect me from her barrage of insults and demands. It was as though I had hardened somehow and was immune to everything. I even did more drugs in those few weeks than I had done in my entire life and I was fine. Now, that Howie has left me bare and vulnerable again, the vest starts slipping off and things start affecting me again.

Stella initiates an argument with me because I wasn't brushing my teeth in the bathroom. What does it matter where I brush my teeth, as long as I brush my teeth? Whenever I tell Howie how much Stella hates me he says I'm being silly in a patronising-teacher kind of way. Or like a nursery supervisor who isn't allowed to say 'naughty' and has to say 'silly' instead.

"Come on Chuck," he says, handing me a spliff so I'll shut up talking about Stella. "No one gets along with their parents."

"Ezra does!" I always say, because Ezra's family would be the epitome of perfection, if Ezra weren't such a jug-head like me. "And you did."

"That's the point, you did too, we all did. Some of us carry on and some of us don't."

I'll calm down as the joint relaxes me, and Howie will put *Velvet Underground* on the old Sony CD player and all my problems with Stella are forgotten.

Until I get back home and nothing has changed.

Even Alice and I are become increasingly detached, more so than usual. I don't even bother asking what she's doing on the stairs at two o' clock in the morning. I don't care anymore. Don't care that she understands James Joyce and I don't, or that she's a genius and my brain hardly even functions properly anymore.

The more distanced I become from Stella and Alice, the closer to each other they become. Where before I used to take my earphones out to

DRIPFEED

hear what they were saying in the hall outside my room, I now turn the volume up and let them get on with it. I just don't know what Alice sees in Stella, or how she could possibly stand more than thirty seconds of her company. The word 'killjoy' was possibly invented for Stella. It's not this house that is draining my happiness, it's Stella. Stella is the driving force that bleeds me dry. How could I have thought, for one minute, that something as inanimate as a house could have the power to render me this morose?

Then one Friday I steal a bag of sweets from Hamley's and instead of being dragged back inside by the heavy security guards, I am punished in some other divine way. Even though God and I gave up on each other a long time ago and I am now atheist, I feel only He could be responsible for what constitutes the rest of my day.

    First of all I am caught out at London Bridge station for having a *child* travel card and am forced to hand over twenty pounds that I really don't have. Then, due to the questioning, fining and ticket-issuing, I miss my train and have to spend the next thirty minutes praying the man tottering dangerously on the wrong side of the yellow line doesn't fall onto the track, thus delaying me further. Just when I think it can't possibly get any worse, I get home and find Howie has cancelled on me; Ezra doesn't want to be my second choice, and Chavez is off somewhere, drunkenly entertaining her new girlfriend. So I take some of the coke I took from Stewie's endless supply, and empty the entire bag onto an old text book, where I then proceed to shove the entire lot up my nose. First and foremost, this is not a suicide attempt – subconsciously or otherwise – I am genuinely trying to block Stella and Howie and Chavez, and all the other people I hate, out of my mind, and the only way I know how is by taking whatever narcotic I have in my possession.

The doctors say it's becoming quite clear I have a problem and should either be institutionalised in the dreaded day-care centre, or stuck on a conveyer belt in rehab. Either way, I need help!

I don't even know I've OD'd until the familiar feelings of heart-beating-out-of-chest and brain-detaching-itself-from-body kick in and I'm spazzing out on the floor again. This time it's Howie who finds me; he came round to apologise for tonight's cancellation. Alice opened the door, amazed at this…man. He came upstairs, knocked on the bedroom door, which was obviously mine, '*DO NOT ENTER*' sign on the door and tantalising aroma of incense and opium leaking from underneath. He didn't bother waiting for a response, just barged right in with a rehearsed apology. Howie has seen enough girls OD in his life and career not to overreact, clutching at my head, screaming for help, killing me with his concern. He takes his jacket off and puts it under my head – I later ask why he didn't just grab a pillow, since we were in my *bed*room and all.

DRIPFEED

Then he calls for Stella, who goes into caring mother mode again, leaving Howie wondering how anyone could possibly hate this woman – least of all me.

"Chuck darling," she screams. "Not again. I thought we were over this. Why?" What she is saying is very clear to me, albeit far-away sounding as if I'm under water. This is what OD'ing does, it takes me far away – metaphorically speaking – to where I can hear everything everyone is saying, but muffled, as if I'm eavesdropping from the other side of a door.

When I wake up an old Asian man in a white coat is standing over my bed with a clipboard. I instantly recognise him as the man always present whenever I end up here.

"Charlotte," he begins. "Why are you always here? Is there something you like about this place? Perhaps it's one of the young doctors?"

"No," I say weakly through the mass of wires and tubes and drips and whatnot.

"Then what – you want to harm yourself?"

"It was an accident," I say trying to twist away from him, finding the tangle of wires preventing me from doing so.

"It's always an accident with you, isn't it?" Snaps Stella from a chair by the door. "How many times have we been here this summer? Not even three months! Since when did you become such a junky?"

I half-expect the nice Asian doctor to jump to my defence, but alas he remains over the bed with the clipboard. He reaches down, searching my eyes with a torch, my ears, my mouth, my nose.

"Have you ever considered talking to someone?" he asks, lifting up my arm, shaking his head at the sheer amount of track marks along its inner surface; even I didn't know I shot that much. "Carry on like this and your veins are going to collapse. And your septum," he adds as an afterthought.

Stella gasps. "Veins!" she shoots me a poisonous look. "Who are you?"

"Who are you?" I manage. "Forget to take your Valium this morning?" The doctor raises an eyebrow.

"I'm keeping you in for observation," he declares. "You could do with the rest."

When the doctor leaves Stella hisses at me from her position on the chair; legs crossed, blood-red talons drumming the padded armrest. "Cocaine! Heroin! Honestly. You must really hate me –" finally, she's catching on. "- You want all these doctors thinking I don't know how to raise my own child? Well, at least you finally got what you wanted; all the attention is finally on you. Don't worry about me, I'm only the one who has to clean all this shit up. I'm only the one whose money you've been using to buy all this crap. You said last time was the last time. You said you'd never touch the stuff again, but here we are, *again*. I don't know why I'm surprised anymore.

DRIPFEED

Coming home at all hours of the morning, room smelling of incense – what are you, Buddha? And *boys*. I thought that boy you always brought home was gay, well, now that I've been privy to another of your conquests I can't be too sure, can I? Where did I go wrong with you? Why can't you be more like Alice? Why are you always the one to disappoint me – to disappoint everyone? No wonder your father left you, he was probably sick of all this. And who could blame him? You probably want to end up like one of the characters in those books you're always reading, or the films and music you're into – you think I don't know. *Confessions of a Trickbaby*, and I don't even want to know what that one's about."

"Are you quite finished?" I ask, in response to Stella's dull soliloquy. "There's no one here, Stella, so who are you performing to?"

"Oh Charlotte." I don't even bother reminding her that I don't like that name, that she couldn't have chosen a worse name for me, that for the last fucking time, my name is CHUCK! Instead I close my eyes and wait for her to get out, where she'll go and tell her friends about her stressful daughter. Yes! The one who's making her anxiety attacks worse. The very same daughter who is causing her so much physical pain that she's being forced to pop more and more of those tiny white sleeping pills to escape it. She'll use me as her excuse, to explain away the empty bottles in the recycling bin, or the slurred, drunken voice on the phone. Once again I'll be blamed for the heart attack she's giving herself.

Lami Okrekson

Why am I like this? It was either this – the inbetweener, the junky, the dark and weird teenage delinquent – or the pregnant-with-four-kids-and-friendless slut, who occasionally puffs the magic dragon and then gets kicked on the face by her drunken boyfriend. I could have been one of those girls, twice removed from my perfectly behaved grandparents, the kind of girl who gets kicked out of home and ends up in a hostel, or some scummy government housing project; the kind of silent junky hiding the scars behind piles of Pampers and Talcum Powder. At least I don't try to hide this shit behind anything.

I could have always been one of the brown-wearing social retards no one knows anything about. The kind of girls who comb their long, dirty, brown hair in front of their faces and wear sweaters that are too big for them, the kind who read James Joyce – and get it; in other words, I *could* have ended up like Alice. Either way, any one of the three alternatives would have led me here, to this hospital bed that Alice will, no doubt, be gracing before she is safely out of her teens and able to see the world for what it really is, not some giant, all-consuming, corporate machine.

I think of all the things I will do when I get out of here, things that Stella will be thoroughly overjoyed by. Perhaps I *will* go to the Hayward gallery with Ezra, or by myself for that matter, who says I need other people to have fun. Or maybe I won't, maybe I'll just lay, inert, on the floor, moving only to take a shit or a hit. Maybe I won't even

DRIPFEED

shower; I'll just lay stinking in my own sweaty sheets practically begging for the blackness.

Howie visits me in the hospital, being in a band constitutes as jobless so he has no money to buy me flowers. He says he bought grapes but got hungry and ate them on the tube. What do I care – this room looks like a vineyard exploded all over it anyway. One more packet of grapes would have tipped it over the edge.

Howie is sullen, which isn't unusual for an indie musician, but he is more sullen than usual.

"Why'd you do it?" He asks quietly. "Was it because I said I couldn't go out? Because if it is, that's crazy. I told you, I had to practice with the band."

This is the most I've heard him say in one breath. "No!" I lie. "Like I told the doctors, it was an accident. I didn't even know I took that much."

"You took a whole bag," he points out.

"So sue me," I say, exasperatedly mimicking Eminem, for whom I used to harbour the most intense adoration.

"You do too much of that anyway," Howie continues. "You do more than me, and I'm trying to quit."

"So what are you saying," I'm looking for an argument now, now that the sedatives are starting to wear off. "That I'm a bad influence? That you'd be better of without me?"

"I didn't say that," he defends. "I just said that you do too much of that stuff. If you don't stop you're going to end up like Pete Doherty, or worse, like every other dead junky.'

"So I'm a junky now?"

"The way you do all that shit, you must be. You don't even know where it comes from half the time, as long as it gets you high."

"Why are we talking about me? Can't you find anything else to talk about?"

"I thought you'd be happy! I thought you liked being the centre of attention. That's why you did this, isn't it? That's why you do all of it. You want people talking about you, to you; about how fucked-up you are, how they're glad they're not you but how much they wanna be your friend. Do you know how many crack heads would love to supply you? Do you even know how much money they'd make off you? You're a fucking gold-mine – where'd you get it anyway, since you hate your mum so much, you can't still be taking her money?"

This is our first argument. "If it bothers you that much, FUCK OFF!" I shout.
The door is open and the nurses outside, arranging flowers or whatever shoots us deadly looks. How dare we use such prolific expletives in a public place – least of all a place where sick children are being healed? "Fuck you then," Howie says before leaving. Now I wish he had brought flowers, then I could throw them at the wall like some drama-queen, vase and all.

Apart from Stella, Howie was my only visitor. My friends have no use for me here, not when my

DRIPFEED

vein space is being taken up by IV's and drips, and my nose and throat space by tubes of oxygen. Why can't they just fix me here?

When I get back home five days later, Alice has gone to some summer camp in the American countryside. This is how far away Stella will send her precious daughter to protect her from my bad influence.

    Although I dislike Alice almost as much as I dislike Stella – for being smarter than me, prettier than I was at that age, in a kind of trash, grungy way – her absence is greatly missed. This is how it always goes: I hate someone so much that they are eventually forced to take my advice and fuck off. Then, when they've gone, and I'm standing in the space they used to occupy, I realise that I kind of miss them. Whether it's Belle and her condescending bullshit, or Alice and her über-intellegence, it's all the same.

Chapter 6

I am lying on Howie's bed smoking a Marlboro, having just spent the last few hours 'making up.' Conveniently, Howie has a mini-fridge in his room, so in addition to the Marlboro, I am also sipping from a Budweiser bottle while Howie listens to the *Stone Roses*, air-drumming with customised sticks. Even though Howie practically ripped me to shreds for doing too much junk and accidentally OD'ing, my veins are still tender from a hit he gave me two hours ago, and I'm still feeling light-headed from the amyl nitrates we popped earlier. Not that I mind, but for someone trying to crack the habit, Howie is hardly the model candidate. And he was worried about me turning into Pete Doherty on my own.

Soon, we move into the living room where the entire band, amongst others, have gathered. I take in this motley crew, a bunch of hippie losers with long hair and bare feet.

"So I hear you OD'd," Stewie says, like I should be proud of it. "

Yeah," I say, not wanting to talk about it in the open amongst all these people, most of whom I don't even know. Howie shoots Stewie a look that says *shut the fuck up or else.* And Stewie shuts up. He – the skinny lead singer – is no match for Howie, slightly beefy drummer-guy. This feels like the first time anyone has ever stood up for me.

DRIPFEED

We spend the next few hours drinking the fridge dry of all its alcohol. The boys debate over the loss of quality in music from then and now.

"Look at all these Boy bands," Justin (lead guitarist) points out. Boy bands are the teeny-bopper bands like *McFly* or *Busted*, the kind of band your thirteen year old sister is supposed to like. These are the shambolic bands of the twenty-first century, the ones taken up the sofas of *Popworld* when it should really be *Basement* up there declaring their love for musical geniuses like Bob Dylan and Bruce Springsteen.

"You're no one if you don't know the *Beatles*," Howie adds. "Boy bands make me sick."

"If they're Boy bands, what are you?" I ask.

Howie and Stewie jump up on the coffee table, knocking some green on the floor, playing air-guitar. "We're a man band," Howie shouts. As if to solidify their point, they go over to the battered old Sony, and put *Sergeant Peppers Lonely Hearts Club Band* on. All the formerly-stoned hippie-types jump up and start swaying and moshing to music that really shouldn't be moshed to. All of *Basement* are up there, on sofas and tables, jumping around like Jack-in-the-box and dripping ash all over the carpet. All of *Basement* except for Justin, who sits coolly smoking a joint, too cool to get involved in the drunken antics of his peers. Justin, unlike Howie, is the kind of man who will say one sentence, that packs such a punch he can remain silent for the rest of the evening and no one will even forget he's there. I watch him without letting him see I'm watching. I make sure there's always a crowd of sweaty stoners in between us before I allow my eyes to fall on his stoned, relaxed face. He is wearing shades, even though we're inside and it's night outside. I don't know if he sees me watching, in fact, I don't even care. I light another Marlboro and look longingly at the cocaine in the middle of the table. So tempted am I, to unsnap the baggie and sniff to my hearts content. I resist the temptation though, purely because this is the only thing that will bring Howie down from that table of happiness, my inability to stay on the right side of that line. My problem is that not only do I cross the line, I go so far over it I can't even see it anymore.

I end up staying over at Howie's, something I've been doing a lot recently. It keeps me away from Stella, keeps me from being alone, sitting in my room doing lines and sniffing paint off an old t-shirt that is pretty much saturated by now. Of course it doesn't keep me off the drugs altogether, that would be asking too much from a group of twenty-something year old bandsters with nothing but their music and their mammoth opium addictions to sustain them.

Howie keeps me up all night going back over the debate about the musical quality of the twenty-first century, assuming that – because I remained silent during the said debate – I am in favour of musical ablutions such as *Busted, McFly* and the late *Noise Next Door*. I am kept up half

DRIPFEED

the night – which is actually half the morning – defending myself and my taste in music.

We get up at four the next afternoon, which is also another of our little occurrences, and view everyone in their bleary-eyed, hungover bloatedness.

Before I leave for home I am introduced to a woman who appears to have materialised from nowhere. I am sure I didn't see her last night and it soon becomes clear she spent *her* night inside Justin's room. This woman is how I imagine Alice will look when she grows up: shabby and stragglylooking, knotty hair all in her face, wearing a thick grey jumper that looks about ten sizes too big for her. She is exactly the kind of social retard I have tried so hard not to become.

I don't go straight home when Howie drops me off at the train station, I go instead to Waterloo and stand on the bridge looking at the water and contemplating jumping in – not to drown, but because once again, I am thinking how enticing the dirty brown water looks. Even though I'd probably be eaten alive by the seven different species of piranha in there, it's cool and tempting and up here on the bridge is so hot and sticky. I don't spend a long time here, just enough to be considered a casual water gazer by the other casual water-gazers – probably also contemplating the jump.
I think I spot Diane amongst the suited-and-booted, remembering her saying something about her and a law firm in Westminster. I count the

number of fat-ankle women to walk past me, the select disproportionate few whom Ezra and I harbour a secret admiration for. I wish Ezra were here now, to point at the ugly people with me and laugh.

A skinny woman in a black suit, talking on a mobile and walking too fast, bangs into a lamp-post and I suppress the desire to burst into fits of that explosive, hysterical laughter I can't control. I can't though, I am alone here and to laugh alone on this Bridge would be like wearing a strait jacket on Oxford Street and singing *The Wheels on The Bus go Round and Round.* I instead redirect my laughter at the River and let it pass.

The house is empty and silent when I get back. No Stella here asking what time I call it. Saying things like, 'you were out doing *drugs* I take it? Didn't you learn from last time?' Stressing that other 'D' word, reverting back to the posh middle-classed-ness that was hers before she threw it away and decided she wanted the fast, reckless life (this I know from eavesdropping on her phone calls). There is no reason for Stella to be here, since Alice isn't. Stella doesn't need to hang around entertaining her, or warming up microwave dinners for her, even though I'm sure Alice is more than capable of doing that herself.

Since my only two options here are to get high or get some sleep, I go for the latter. I've pretty much exhausted my supply anyway, and it wouldn't do for Stella to come back and find me spazzing out on the floor again – days after being

DRIPFEED

hospitalised due to yet another of my overdoses, or worse, dead.

Due to my sleeping most of the day away, I am not even remotely tired and, as a result of this, start to do something entirely uncharacteristic of me. I go out into the garden and proceed to water all the dead-looking plants back to life. I say 'start to' because that is as far as I get. I water an apple tree, get bored, and pour the rest of the water on the ground. I catch my nosy neighbour reprimanding me silently from her window; I am wasting water at a time where water is so precious. How dare I be so fucking insensitive?

Even though I didn't feel tired when I tried to nourish all those dead, rotting plants, all that sleep is having its counter-productive effects on me again, and I crawl up the stairs trying to stop my head from rolling off my neck and back down away from me. I had no idea a full-time relationship could be so consuming. I fall onto my bed fully-clothed, and dream of the red attacking lips. Somehow, this dream isn't as scary as I once thought. They're just lips; I'll get up later and carry on my life as normal with or without the bodiless lips. After that the dreams stop.

Chapter 7

Howie asks me to go on a road-trip with him. By 'road trip,' he actually means, as far North as his car will allow, and then back round, the long way. In other words, a round trip of the UK – or as long as it takes to get bored, realise other, more pressing engagements, blah, blah, blah. I say yes, of course. I'm on a hiatus from education anyway, no job, no immediate commitments, what difference will it make to anyone if I just disappear for a couple of days? Lazing around in a car is no different to lazing around in my room, at least this way I'll be moving, I'll get a chance to see the scenery instead of being stationary and inert.

We leave immediately, me showing up at his flat with two duffle bags of clothes and provisions, lighting up a Marlboro while Howie stares at the luggage saying, we're not going back-packing in India you know, they do have shops outside of London.

The farewell ceremony at Howie's is exactly like the one I got at home. Stella waved a drunken hand in my direction. "If this is what you want, I can't stop you," she had said, like I told her I was going to fight on the front line in Iraq. Do your duty if you will but don't come crying to me when your legs get blown off. She didn't even ask when I'd be back, where exactly I'd be staying, just who this Howie was anyway – the usual things a normal mother would. She just waved me on,

DRIPFEED

told me to go – the sooner the better as far as she was concerned.

Back at Howie's flat he gets a nod from Stewie and an inaudible mumble from the woman in the grey sweater. We lug my bags down three flights of stairs, because the lift broke, and chuck the stuff into Howie's car.
    Four and a half hours later, arriving in Leeds, I start to think that maybe this wasn't such a good idea. For one, the heat inside the car is unbearable – even with the windows open. This global warming thing must really be taking off. A couple of years ago thirty degrees was as hot as it got. Now thirty-five is the benchmark, the bar set for a boiling hot summer. Summer in England didn't used to be like this, before countless deodorant cans and car exhausts, summer used to be twenty-five degrees if you were lucky, and sixteen if you weren't.

We had planned to live out of the car for this little trip, but as we'd probably be fried alive in our own sweat, we decide against it. Combined, all we can afford is a tiny room in a grotty-looking bed 'n' breakfast, except they don't even serve breakfast so it's just bed 'n' see-how-many-cockroaches-you-can-spot.
    Inside, I feel like staying in the car would have been a lot cooler. The room is probably hotter than the sun. I thank God I don't wear make-up, because it'd probably be dripping all over the floor by now. There is, of course, no air-

conditioning in here; the windows only open slightly, which lets in flies and spiders, but not much air. And the bed looks like it was lifted from some military base. I bet if I look close enough I'll see *UK ARMY* branded on the side.

"What do you think?" Howie looks hopeful. Hoping that I'm too excited to notice what a shit-hole this is.

"It's nice." I try to sound bright, and inject some tone into my voice, but it comes out dry. Either way it pleases Howie.

Howie wants to go to a pub; since we're in Leeds we might as well make the most of all the cheap beer and student hang-outs. I feel strange about leaving our stuff here in the room though. It's only stuff, but the woman who owns this place – some weird Mexican who seems so out-of-place here in Northern England – looks like she wouldn't mind using her spare set to get in here and have a good poke around. Howie doesn't mind; naturally.

"Fuck it," he says. "It's only clothes." It's not only clothes to me, he doesn't seem to realise it's my life in there. I don't bother telling him this; he'd only say why'd you bring it then?

We find a pub, a student bar that's cheaper than the Wetherspoon's across from the B&B, and is surprisingly packed for four in the afternoon. The girl behind the bar lets us off; she thinks we are students who have forgotten their student identification. I could see myself living here.

DRIPFEED

"How's Stella?" Howie asks. "Still crazy?" It's funny how, even though *I'm* allowed to bitch and moan about how much I hate Stella, it still feels weird to hear other people say it. Not that I care, really, but I find myself getting pissed off, really pissed off, like, if I had hackles they'd definitely be raised. I laugh it off though.

"Yeah. Still psycho bitch."

"What's she done this time?" Howie gets serious all of a sudden; it's as if, by admitting to him that she's crazy, I have revealed some deeper, darker side to myself.

"Same as usual: arguing, nit-picking, accusing. You name it."

"Why don't you just stay at ours?" Why don't I? It would be a million times better than living in the constant battle between suicide and carrying on. It would take me away from everything I'm dying to get away from anyway; so why not? I would feel guilty, about leaving Alice behind. As much as we don't get on, I wouldn't want to leave her there, not yet anyway. Who knows, maybe Stella would switch – although I hardly see that happening. Alice will always be the golden child, the one with the straight A's, the one who skips a couple of years and goes straight to Oxford. And even if she doesn't, even if she rock-bottoms it out and lands on her laurels in a crack-house shooting heroin into her eyeballs, she'll still be on that pedestal of infinite greatness. She'll still be the one who could have been, would have been, if life hadn't got in the way. No matter what Alice does, whenever, she'll always be better than me.

"Well?" Prompts Howie, bringing me back from wherever it is that I went. "Why don't you just stay at ours?"

"You've got too much to think about. The band, a job, paying the rent. And besides, you can't afford me, I'd eat too much!"

"I thought heroin addicts were supposed to *lose* their appetites?"

"Exactly," I say. "Then I'm not addicted am I?" Neither of us say anything, about the fact that – in all actuality – I probably *am* addicted, that I'm so skinny I could give Kate Moss a run for her money, that the real reason I can't stay in that opium den is because there'd be too much temptation to resist. I'd die. I'd get so addicted that I would just die, albeit happy and stoned; a death is a death is a death, after all.

I like this place, whoever said people up North were happiest had it right. Although this is only one bar in one city in one section, it is clear to me that the people here aren't so uptight and highly strung all the time, or talking so animatedly on mobile phones that they bang into lampposts, get up, and carry on with that impending angina. Even though all the people in here are broker-than-broke students drinking away their student loans and overdrafts, they seem so laid back about it. I could live here and not even need any of that manmade crap to sustain me.

DRIPFEED

After the pub we walk around Leeds, close to our bed 'n' breakfast so we don't get lost. Howie knows a man in Manchester, so we're apparently going there tomorrow.

"Why didn't we just go there first? It's closer to London."

Howie just shrugs nonchalantly.

The night spent in that B&B was perhaps the worst night I have had in my life. I've shared bedrooms with cockroaches in the past; I've seen a lot worse than the inside of a dodgy bed 'n' breakfast – and I didn't have anyone to share my fears with then. The problem then, is me. I've grown too used to clean bedrooms and white porcelain bathtubs. Thought of blood-stained toilet bowls and cockroaches don't tend to fill my thoughts everyday. The first one appears out of nowhere. It's too hot to sleep and I'm lying on my back staring at the wall. I blink and there it is, huge and black, staring at me with eyes I can't see. I've never been much of a screamer – I've been desensitized by too many creepy-crawlies to be that shocked by them – but this is an exception. Although I knew the likelihood of seeing cockroaches here was high anyway, I didn't *really* expect it. That, or I thought I'd be asleep by the time they hit, too tired to feel them crawling their way across my face.

The scream isn't loud enough to wake Howie, or bring the Mexican lady in from her ground floor bedroom, and I am forced to endure this alone.

Lami Okrekson

As quickly as the first one appeared, it disappears and others start following suit. It is dark, but the curtains are practically see-through and there is a street lamp right outside the window. Anyone would have thought the light would be enough to deter them. I can hear them but I can't always see them. They sound like moths flying into a foam ceiling, crackly and dry against the peeling paint and woodchip. I hear them in stereo surround sound. They are all around me, above and below. I would like to take Howie's keys and go sleep in the car, but then I'd have to put my feet on the floor and who knows what could be lurking down there. The cockroaches are making me so edgy. If only I could see them, then I wouldn't have to keep lifting up the covers to make sure they didn't get under there. I wouldn't have to keep brushing my arms and legs down to check they weren't on me. I wouldn't be hiding, sweating, under a winter blanket in twenty-five degrees of heat.

The final straw comes when a cockroach actually appears on Howie's chest. He brushes it off in his sleep and it disappears under the bed. But if that one managed to get up here, more will follow. Knowing I will never fall asleep, with all these roaches running around with God knows what – rats and mice probably, I reach over into my night bag and take out my spray-on deodorant. Slipping my t-shirt off over my head I saturate it with the deodorant and lean back to inhale the fumes. Although the effect is short-lived, it lasts long enough to knock me out and send me into a

DRIPFEED

deep sleep. I wake up in the morning before Howie, with the t-shirt still over my face, glad that I woke up first.

In the sunlight the roaches seem to have disappeared and the room is still and silent. It's funny how things always look better in the morning and I wonder if I was really under siege last night or if my mind was just playing tricks on me. Either way I'll be glad to get out of this place. In the cold, harsh light of day, Leeds doesn't look so good anymore.

Howie wakes up and we check out, hitting the road again. I hope to God we never have to sleep in another room like that.

We head down to Manchester, where Howie knows the guy.

"What did you think of Leeds?" Howie asks.

"It was alright, if you don't count all the roaches and spiders."

"What roaches?"

"The ones that invaded our room last night."

"I didn't see any."

Of course not. "You were asleep," I say. "So who is this man in Manchester anyway?"

"Some guy I was in a band with once. He went into rehab and we all split."

"Oh!" I raise my eyebrows.

"What?" Howie asks.

"Nothing. Did it work out, the rehab I mean?"

"Nah, I don't think it ever does. Absence makes the heart grow fonder and all that. He told them he was fine, I think he even believed it – cos they let him out, but when he came out he was back. I haven't seen him since before he went in, but I heard he's back on the smack."

"Oh."

"And don't go getting any ideas." Howie says. "I don't want you to OD again."

I feel like a child. Maybe I will OD again just to prove them right and make them feel good about themselves for the half hour it takes to phone an ambulance and have me carted off back to the emergency room. This time it might not be drips and IV's, it might be strait jackets and therapy. It might be a mental institution with visits on the weekend. "I won't," is all I say.

"What are you thinking?" Howie asks without taking his eyes off the road.

"Nothing you'd wanna hear." I light a cigarette with one of Howie's many lighters and breathe the smoke out of the open car window. With the window down, the cigarette in my hand, and my bare feet hanging out of the window, I feel like I should be in a movie, or rather, I could lift Geena Davis out of Susan Sarandon's nineteen sixty-six Thunderbird and take her place. Always the passenger, never the driver.

"I wish I could take a picture of you like that," Howie says, taking his eyes off the road for a second. I ignore him and flick the cigarette butt out of the window lighting up another one.

DRIPFEED

"I wonder if it's illegal to stick your feet out of the window of a moving vehicle," I say out loud. Howie says nothing.

Halfway between Leeds and Manchester, I find an old bottle of rum in the glove compartment. Howie and I down the entire bottle and fall asleep in a shallow ditch in the middle of a field. Before we fall asleep we throw the empty bottle in a river – fucking nature up like us – and smoke the last of my Marlboros. "Fuck! Fuck! Fuck!" Howie shouts when we wake up, still drunk, a few hours later. Some birds fly over, other than that it's silent.
"We should sleep out here tonight," I suggest. "It's better than sleeping in the car, or finding another bed 'n' breakfast with cockroaches and fleas."
"Yeah." Howie is a champion lightweight and falls asleep instantly. I, on the other hand, am left alone, again. I remember that *field mice* are called *field mice* for a reason, and a field full of mice is, in some respects, worse than a room full of roaches. Cockroaches don't bite.
This time I don't even have the spray can within my reach; I'd have to go back to the car – and who knows if I'd make it back here in the dark. I reach for the packet of Marlboro's before realising the empty box can't help me. Now that Howie's asleep and I'm alone again, the prospect of spending the night alone in an open field does not seem as appealing as it did a few hours ago. Aside from the mice, there could be other

creatures in here: snakes, poisonous spiders, foxes, coyotes, wolves!

I stop with the crazy thoughts for a while and look at the sky. I so rarely get to do this in London; too much pollution, not enough time, whatever. The stars are out. I wish I knew what to look for, then I might spot Orion's Belt or a shooting star. As it is, half of the bright lights I think are stars are probably just aeroplanes, and as for *Orion's Belt*, I have more chance of spotting E.T.

I really need to take a piss, but I don't want to go out into the wilderness and get mangled by a couple of bored, hungry hyenas. Instead, I cross my legs and hold it till morning.

"This feels good," Howie says, back on the road, back on the way to Manchester. It's a surprise the car was still there when we woke up.

"What?" I say. "Not being able to brush your teeth, or take a piss in a toilet?"

"No. This! All the fucking nature and stuff. We should go camping."

"Yeah," I say.

It has only been a few hours since my last cigarette, but already I'm feeling the lacking in my blood without the nicotine there to supplement it. I can't wait until we hit Manchester so I can get some more cigarettes and stock up some quality cocaine from this crack head Howie wants to see. Right now, I don't give a fuck about Howie, about OD'ing, about dying even. I haven't done anything

DRIPFEED

harder than half a can of Sure deodorant since we left almost two days ago. I want some class A's and I want them now!

"Breakfast?" Howie suggests.

"No!" I say, still thinking about the cocaine I'll have some when we get to Manchester. Fuck that even! All I want is a nice fat needle and some time to forget about the roaches and the rats and the coyotes and the hyenas. Right now, I want to get so smashed that I can't even remember my own name.

"You *don't* want breakfast?" Howie is saying.

"Oh. Yeah. I thought you said something else."

Howie's probably thinking, what the fuck rhymes with 'breakfast' – how could she think I said something else? He doesn't say any of this; he just carries on driving towards a MacDonald's on the motorway, checking the tank, smiling because it is half full.

We don't find a MacDonald's on the motorway but come across a tiny *Little Chef*. The place is deserted, and in this heat, I half expect to see tumbleweed rolling by. The station has a toilet and a phone box outside it. It's too eerie, too quiet. It reminds me of every other horror movie involving a deserted petrol station: *Jeepers Creepers, The Hitcher*. They both involved some shack of a petrol station out on the middle of nowhere.

Lami Okrekson

We go inside where one woman in a dirty uniform is standing behind the counter smoking a cigarette. The cravings come back and I go over to a cigarette machine, which is empty. Fuck! When I get back to the counter Howie has two cups of coffee. I feel dirty about drinking coffee when I haven't even brushed my teeth. Coffee stains.

You'd think a woman who had been standing alone behind a counter all day would be glad for the company of two paying customers. You'd think she would then do as much as she could to ensure the return of those two customers. Not this woman. This woman takes our order – of bacon and egg sandwiches – to the back and looks at us as if to say, don't blame me, I'm just the waitress.

At a table Howie says. "*Oceans Eleven* came on a few nights ago."

"Which one?" I ask.

"The one with George Clooney. Did you watch it?"

"Obviously not." Idiot! "Otherwise I would have known which one it was, wouldn't I?"

"You should have watched it. It was fucking class, best film ever."

"Yeah, I suppose."

"I thought you said you didn't see it?" Howie asks.

"I've seen it before. That man gets on my nerves though, the one with the British accent. What's the point of that? It sounds so fake."

DRIPFEED

"Nah," Howie says. "That just makes it better. He's a fucking genius, he makes the film funnier."

"There was no point of that accent," I continue. "It's just like every other American who does a British accent; it sounds fake. It sounds like they're taking the piss, or else that's how they think all British people speak."

"What about when British people do an American accent then? Like Minnie Driver or Catherine Zeta-Jones?"

"That's different," I say. "It's not so obvious. It doesn't sound like a piss take."

"I didn't know it offended you so much," Howie says.

"It doesn't. I just don't know why Don Cheadle had to do the accent."

Howie sips from the coffee cup, grimacing at the heat or the taste. "But it's convincing, so what's the problem?" Why can't the food just hurry up and come so this conversation can be over and done with? I look towards the counter, where the woman is still smoking an endless chain of cigarettes and looking at a magazine.

"Yeah it's convincing, *I* thought he was British at first, but the accent is so out of place in that film, I mean, what would a common Brit be doing amongst America's top cat-burglars? It doesn't make sense."

Howie thinks for a moment. "It's a film; it doesn't have to make sense. Without Cheadle, the film wouldn't have been so –" he struggles for a word.

"- Boring? Stupid? Pointless?"

"I thought you said you liked it?"

"Whatever. There was no need for that accent. It's an American film, if they wanted British people they should have gotten British people."

Howie is getting annoyed; he has the pained expression on his face of someone who is trying hard not to hit someone. "Okay fine, he says. "Then what about Vincent Gallo in *Confessions*? What about his accent?"

"That was different," I say, defending my favourite movie. "They were *in Mexico*. He was Mexican. He's hardly gonna have an American accent is he?"

"Exactly! And Don Cheadle was British. He's hardly gonna have an America accent either."

"Oh whatever," I say.

The food has finally arrived and is sitting, growing cold, on the counter. The woman in the dirty uniform is making no effort to bring it over to us; in fact, she still hasn't looked up from her magazine – not even to note that her latest cigarette has turned to an ashen mess in her hand.

"I'll get it," Howie says, noting my disgusted face. We eat the cold, greasy bacon and egg sandwiches in silence. We have exhausted ourselves. We don't usually talk this much; our conversations usually follow the dull, monosyllabic patterns of people trying to make

DRIPFEED

small talk. How could one topic have cleaned us out like this?

Back on the road, Howie says. "We're nearly there."
"Oh," I say.
Stan, the man from Manchester, is exactly the junky I hoped for and expected him to be. I almost cry when I see this emaciated, drunk-looking, specimen of man standing there in a dirty white vest. His dirty blonde hair matches the vest and he is smoking a cigarette. Cigarette! I don't care if they're B&H, I don't even care if they're Park Road. This man has cigarettes and I am staying at his house. For now, this emaciated, heroin-addict is God.
"Stan!" Howie exclaims.
"Howie!" Stan exclaims. If Stan weren't so skinny Howie probably would have hugged him. As it stands, Stan is probably skinnier than me, and a hug from Howie would have shattered what little of his bones remain.

The first thing I do when I get inside the flat is to locate the packet of cigarettes – which happen to be Silk Cut – from the table, and light one with a match in a box next to it. I do not care that this isn't my house, that I should really have asked first before helping myself. I inhale deeply and smile as the nicotine flows through my veins. There is also a bag of coke on the table, Howie and Stan are talking in the kitchen, and I am sure Stan wouldn't miss one tiny drop. Even though stealing his drugs would be much worse than stealing his cigarettes, he's a crack head, 'share and share alike,' right? Before I have time to decide whether or not to take the coke, Howie and Stan come back in.

"And who might you be?" Stan asks.

"Chuck."

"Nice to meet you, Chuck," he extends a hand, which I take. "Help yourself." He motions to the bag on the table. I don't need telling twice. I can feel Howie's eyes burning a hole in the back of my head, trying to melt that bag of cocaine with his laser-vision before I have the chance to get at it. I empty a little bit onto the table and sort it into thin white lines. "It's not gold dust you know," says Stan. "You can do more than that. If your old man doesn't mind, that is."

"You are my angel," I say to him.

I do the first two lines and then sort another two – bigger this time. After the fourth, I lean back in the chair contented and light a cigarette. After a while Howie rubs a bit of the powder on his gums, it must be that good because he forgets what he told me in the hospital, about 'laying off that shit,' and sorts himself a couple of lines. Stan sits in the chair opposite me, grinning a wide, yellow smile.

Stan must owe Howie a huge favour or something, because we end up spending the next few days in his flat: injecting, snorting, smoking, and joking. The place is grotty; worse even than the bed 'n' breakfast in Leeds – except Stan's place doesn't

DRIPFEED

have cockroaches or rats, which is a surprise considering the sheer amount of dirt in the place.

Stan lets us go two days later, with promises to come back soon. We take the long way home; I buy a carton of Marlboros and Howie buys petrol. The ride home is always quicker than the ride there. I spend most of it asleep. I feel guilty because Howie has no one to share his tiredness with.

Chapter 8

I'm beginning to think Howie and I spend too much time together, not enough time as the people we were before we became one half of a couple. I realise I am seeing less and less of Ezra, I hardly ever see Chavez, and as for my own family: ships passing in the night and all that.

Little things about Howie start pissing me off, like the way he has to spin things around in his fingers all the time, long, thin things, like pens, or forks, or the drum sticks he has to bring with him everywhere we go. The sticks, always there, always getting between us, on the train, in the car, on the table. I don't know why something this small irritates me so much, but I begin to understand about married couples divorcing over the most trivial things, like bad eating habits, or shitting with the door open.

Another thing that is beginning to grate on my nerves is the fact that, although we are always together, we are never alone together. We don't do the whole *movie-and-dinner* thing that most couples our age do, we stay inside at Howie's flat with about fifty other people, smoking, drinking blah, blah, blah. Or we go to mine, sit in my bedroom when Stella's out, smoking pot and listening to *Radiohead.* Our problem is that we are stagnant. We haven't *become* stagnant, we started out like this, immobile, inert, lacking in the initiative that is draining us. I don't know what drew us to each other, I can't remember, to look at

DRIPFEED

us you'd think we were nothing more than distant friends. We don't parade our relationship to the world, hands held, arms swinging, smiling, laughing. Our only smiles are the ones that fix themselves upon our faces when we are too stoned to do anything but lay there and let it happen.

Unsurprisingly, this is where I am now; sitting in a chair with Howie, a bottle of Grolsch fixed to my hand. The woman from the other night is here also, still in that gargantuan grey sweater.

Alice came back from camp this morning, tired and jet-lagged, but still full of eleven-year-old energy. In her absence, I decided to make the effort to be nicer to her. I've watched *Ricki Lake* and *Jerry Springer*, I've seen all those estranged siblings meeting for the first time in years, angry and bitter, having harboured feelings of neglect and abandonment. Stella is no positive influence and I don't want Alice to ever think I abandoned her. Seeing her face this morning reminded me of when she was born. She looked like five years had been knocked off her, she looked like a kid again, not some little scientist. I realised I had missed her, and even bent down to give her a hug – though I didn't have to bend that far considering she is tall for her age, where as I just stand at my just-below-average five four and a half.

"Good times?" I asked. She scrutinized me carefully before answering; no doubt she knew what happened, why she had to be whisked away to a camp that had never before been mentioned in this house.

"Yeah," she said. And somehow I was glad that she said 'yeah' instead of 'yes.' "It was cool, we went canoeing and abseiling and rock climbing..." blah, blah, blah.

After a while I switched off. I could hear her, the undertone of her voice, but the words escaped me and I only caught the recount in snippets and names. "Real oak furniture...John, Bob, Sarah...trees...cowboys..." Then I just stopped trying to listen and just said 'yeah,' when there were gaps in the conversation. Maybe this shit really has fried my brain; before I blocked people out because I could; now I can't help it.

After seeing Alice I phoned Ezra. We talked briefly about me, Howie, Stewie, *and Basement* in general. He told me he was off the drugs, by 'drugs' he meant class A's. He said he found an old magazine that had a picture of Daniella Westbrook and her "nose." "That was nasty," he said. "What if that ever happened to us?" He said 'us' like I was coming off the drugs too, like this was just another of our dual attempts at a healthier life – coming clean and staying clean, without rehab and shock therapy. I didn't know what to say after that, 'yeah well, I'm still shovelling it up my nose like nasal spray,' or, 'oh well; a nose is a nose is a nose.' I just said "Yeah," again, like I agreed, and hung up.

DRIPFEED

Sitting on this dull brown sofa day after day has become less than a monotonous routine, it is just so fucking debilitating; like sleeping too much and becoming bed-ridden, the kind where you don't even want to get up to use the toilet.

I get up and go up the stairs to the bathroom. There is a syringe on the floor with some heroin still in it, and I think 'what the hell?' Like Marilyn Monroe said, "Sometimes *what the hell* is the best answer." I sit on the floor leaning against the bathtub, clench my fist because I don't have a belt or anything, and shoot myself up with this discarded needle. There must have been a lot in the syringe and I know it was too much when the orgasmic effect wears off too quickly and is replaced by the intense itching and a desperate need to vomit. I close my eyes and try to picture the men standing atop Canary Wharf waiting to jump off the edge.

When I open my eyes Howie and Justin are in the bathroom with me. Howie is shaking me and shouting. Justin just stands by the door in shades, smoking a joint, smirking.

"What the fuck!" Howie is shouting. "What the fuck are you doing? What the fuck are you doing?" He keeps repeating the question over and over like that, then he starts crying and I start smiling. Howie gets up, shoves past Justin, and leaves the room. Justin comes over.

"Didn't you OD last week?" He asks.

"I think so." Last week, last night, last month, it's all the same to me now.

"Here," Justin presses the joint he was smoking into my hand, rolling and lighting another when I accept. "You want this don't you?" I still feel a bit weak from the hit I took, like I always do, but I smoke the joint anyway, not caring what will happen to me. We stay like that in the bathroom for ages, smoking our joints and smirking.

When I go back into the room hours later, Howie is hunched over on a chair and the grungy-looking woman is rubbing his back and whispering in his ear. Why bother crying? It's not like we've been together forever, it's not even like he didn't know. We met on a milk carton over a bag of cocaine for fucks sake, what did he expect?

I decide to spend the night here, again. Howie is still downstairs being consoled by the woman in grey, so I just climb into his bed and stare at the ceiling, making shapes out of the markings up there, the way some people do with clouds.

Howie comes in later, when I am still awake. "What is wrong with you?" He asks, sitting on the edge of the bed. "Are you trying to kill yourself?"

"No," I reply. "I was just taking a hit, like we always do."

"Not like we always do," Howie says. "Alone in a bathroom with some random needle you find on the floor. That could have been anyone's."

"So I'll get a blood test," I say, deliberately missing the point.

DRIPFEED

"You're missing the point. Why do you do these things? What are you trying to prove?"

"Nothing. I told you I –" He cuts me off.

"I don't get you, Chuck, and I don't think you should be doing this. Stop taking all this crap, at least stop using it so much."

"Why? I'm not addicted." Howie laughs and I know what he's thinking. Even *I* know I'm addicted, I have been for ages. I blame Ezra, for bringing me into this and then getting out while he still could. I hate him for being able to quit, while I'm left here getting the third degree from my overwrought boyfriend.

"I'm gonna stop with the class A's," Howie says after a while. "You should too."

I could quit if I wanted to. I'm addicted but I'm not dependant. I still get high on heroin; I don't take it to keep the pains of withdrawal away. I don't take it to feel normal. And besides, I'd know if I was too far-gone; when it happens, if it happens – if I become so addicted that I actually want to kill for one more hit – then I'll stop. How hard can it be? The fact is not that I *can't* stop. It's that I don't *want* to stop. I want to carry on fucking shit up with Ezra, and if not with Ezra then with Howie, and if not with Howie then by myself. What's so bad about sitting in my room with the curtains closed, doing lines off an old textbook? What's the difference between doing it with other people and doing it alone? Why couldn't I have just done it once and forgotten about it?

Lami Okrekson

It is impossible to try heroin once, because when you do it for the first time – chasing the dragon because you're scared of addiction and disease – it's horrible. It makes you so sick you swear you will never do it again. But you do it again, because you want to experience that high everyone is always talking about, and the first time didn't count. Then you want to do it again, after that, because it was so nice and even if you don't crave it you still have the memory of it. When you decide to go one step further and inject, you will crave it. They say addiction sets in after just seventy-two hours of use.
    I am different.

Howie is not answering his phone, like I did in the beginning. I start hanging out in Starbucks again. I accidentally screw one of the waiters in there, he bought me a coffee – what was I supposed to do? I think about telling Howie this, as I walk home from the man's bedsit in Thornton Heath. I didn't even know his name, or I did but then I forgot. I dismiss the idea of telling Howie, he'd probably start crying again, and I hate it when men cry in front of me; not that they have to be all macho all the time, but in front of me! That is definitely shit I could do without. I'm glad Howie didn't do it in front of me that time, that he had the decency to go and do it away from me, in front of the grungy-looking woman with all that hair in her face. I wonder what he would say though, or what I would say when he asked why I did it. I'd probably say it was an accident, which it was. I hadn't planned

DRIPFEED

on cheating this early on in the relationship. I hadn't planned on cheating at all.

Back at Howie's flat, my lack of guilty conscience prevents me from feeling any guilt about cheating. He's let me back into his life again, although he's barely talking to me. I keep remembering that one time in the café on the motorway, how much we had to say, even if it was only about a topic that could have seduced anyone. Now we're back at square one, worse than that even – because we are worse off than when we started. We are at square negative fifteen. Fifteen chances to pack up and go home. Fifteen chances to see the world. Fifteen chances to start again.

We are all here as usual, sitting in chairs, on the floor, wherever there is space. As usual I am drinking a warm Grolsch straight out of the bottle. Warm because it is summer and things get hot really quickly, out of the bottle because there aren't any cups anymore.

Warm beer is more acid-tasting than cold beer. It makes my face twitch like when I was just getting used to Stella Artois. Justin appears out of nowhere and switches my warm, flat beer for a cold one. The top has already been taken off and I suppose I should be suspicious of spiking, of Rohypnol – the silent, odourless drug, or worse – LSD, ecstasy crushed up and poured inside. I'd never taste it through all those hops and yeast. I drink it anyway – Justin wouldn't go for open rape, he wouldn't get very far anyway, not with all those people, he'd have to find a way of getting me on my own first.

Justin keeps me in supply of cold beers and spliffs all night. It's as if he's there with an ice-cold bottle the moment the one in my hand goes dull and flat. We don't exchange any words, just the beers. This arrangement is fine with me; I'm mellow right now, too mellow to get myself a cold drink.

At some point during the evening I leave to go to the bathroom. I don't know what I expected to find there, another syringe maybe – to shoot myself up with, whatever. There is no such syringe on the bathroom floor this time, not even a drop of anything to put in it. I feel like crying, let down because I couldn't get high, because Howie brought me to this place and then abandoned me, because Justin is the only one who truly gets what I want. I actually sit on the floor and start to cry, huge, gulping attention-seeking tears. Justin comes in while I am still leaning against the side of the bath crying. He doesn't ask why I'm crying, perhaps he just doesn't care. He stands by the door, smirking in his shades, spliff dangling from his lower lip. Then he comes over and sits beside me on the floor. I make no effort to conceal my tears; I carry on crying as I was before. Neither of us says anything to one another, neither of us has to. Presently, Justin takes a spoon out of his pocket and starts cooking some smack with a lighter. The mere sight of the drug is enough to bring me out of this stupid, little girl-ness and I stop crying long enough to watch him effortlessly

DRIPFEED

cook the heroin on a spoon, soak it into a cigarette filter and draw it into a syringe. I know without asking that the syringe is for me.

Justin smiles at me before pulling my arm towards him and rolling up my sleeve.

Howie must have found me on the floor, knocked-out again, because when I wake up it's after three and he's gone. He's not in his bedroom and I can't see the car from the window. Now I know he saw me, and he's pissed off again because I should have learned my lesson last time. I don't want to spend the night alone and Justin's probably off entertaining grungy-chick, so I leave. I go straight home; it's too dark for any water-gazing.

Night is where bad men like to lurk. The bad men we hear about on the news, or read about in the paper. Ones who take innocent girls like me from bridges late at night. Ones who think they are doing the public a great service by ridding the world of all harlots and whores. Thoughts like this are enough to send me straight home to my bed, where the bad men are nothing more than a shadow in a street lamp.

Chapter 9

I am walking through Oxford Street, at one-thirty in the afternoon, in the height of summer. Hustle and bustle, sweaty bodies jam-packed together on pavements too small to support a nation this big. A face floats past me – and lingers with me long after – a hollow, vulnerable face, where the eyes and lips seem to have taken over. Too big, too much, to compliment a head that small. Shrunken in on itself, it would seem, from years of malnutrition, months of torture and neglect. So alien-like, with a deep quality of sadness surrounding it like a halo.

This face scares me, not because of its seeming absence of human likeness, but because I see a reflection of myself placed on top of it, like tracing paper cartoons. I'll end up there, a hollow, shrunken membrane of my former self. I can't bear it, the thought that I could become so reduced, that I could do so much damage to the inside of my body it could transcend to my face, my first impression, the first thing people will see when they see me. And they'll know, just like I know, what it was that caused so much damage; all those dark circles and gaunt gothica. I could always back out, quit while I'm ahead and save myself the heartache. Stop this thing from spreading me on the bed like it has been. I'd be safe. If only I had the willpower to say 'no!' Correction, 'no' is easy – it's only a word. If only I had the *power* to *want* to say 'no!' The truth is I'm

DRIPFEED

not ready to shake this thing from my bones yet. Who knows, maybe in time I will be. But for now I'm enjoying being spread out, dissected like this. It hurts less this way. This is the piece I love.

Chapter 10

I take to wandering around central London again. Since I have no friends left, since Howie has been blocking me out, I have no one to call except for Chavez. The place I wander most is, quite obviously, Waterloo Bridge. The place contains so much nostalgia, from the days before *Miss Selfridge* and *Basement*.

I must have known Howie would get bored of me, everyone does, Stella hit it on the head when she said, 'that's why your father left you.' Left you! Left me! Everyone leaves me eventually, it is part of the pattern I have been conditioned to accept without question. I so should have seen this coming. The only one who really cares whether I live or die is Justin. Justin who always refills my glass when it is empty. Not Howie, when it should be Howie, but Justin. Weird Justin who always asks me if I just OD'd. Strange and profound Justin who only has to say one word for it to be okay. Justin who should have been on the milk crate instead of him.

And so I find myself going over to Howie's flat when I know Howie will be out and Justin will be in, where I'm free to inhale as much as I want, smoke as much as I want, and not feel guilty about the fact that I don't actually feel guilty.

Justin cares so much that he knows what I want even when I don't. Even when I've done too much and need to go and lay down in Howie's

DRIPFEED

bed, Justin knows that I can still handle some more, that I'm still not over that line yet. Even when I'm so drunk that I've thrown up in the toilet bowl, Justin cares so much that he knows I can still drink some more. He knows when I'm too far gone to go home, and hides me in his room for nights on end. That is how much Justin cares for me; he cares so much that he'd even lie to hide my damage from Howie.

I stop becoming addicted to the narcotics and start becoming addicted to Justin instead. I need him to stay at 'normal.' Even though Howie and I made up again – talked a bit, smoked a bit, fucked a bit – I still keep going over there to see Justin. I need him.

"You want this don't you?" Justin waves a small bag of cocaine in my face. How well he knows me. How caring he is. How much he must love me to keep me in such a constant supply.

Sometimes, when I'm at home laying on my bed and staring at my own foam ceiling, I wonder when I started *needing*. When *it* was just about breaking some rules and having some fun. Doing something the parents would hate. Now the funny part is seeing how long I can go before I *need* to call Justin, to get him over here because Howie wouldn't understand. I am now so addicted to Justin I find it hard to be away from him. And it's not even what he can bring – and he always brings – it's about his hair, his dirty fingernails, the smell of him, the shades he wears to hide his dilated pupils. I am falling in love with all these pieces of him, but not him himself.

I become so dependant on Justin, so consumed by the sheer quantity of him, that the Stella-proof vest comes back. The one Howie ripped off when he left me naked and bare. Stella's bullshit starts bouncing off me again.

I am lying on the ground in the garden listening to *Radiohead* through earphones when Stella comes outside with a woman I have never seen before – although I am stoned up to my eyeballs so what do I know?

"There she is," Stella says as if I'm not there. "I can't be bothered anymore; she's always like this, always lying on the floor listening to this suicide music. She's not well, I think." The woman doesn't say anything, even though I'm looking right at her. I don't blame her, what *can* she say? Stella put her on the spot; the poor bitch probably doesn't even know what to think. She probably thinks she can't agree that she will offend Stella if she does.

I stay lying on the floor while they stand staring at me for ages before going inside to drink coffee – or whatever – and discuss why I'm such a head case. I stay where I am, I like being this close to the ground where I can hear the ants running around by my face. I don't care what the neighbours think of this, but I do wonder if they think of this.

DRIPFEED

Naturally, Justin and I start sleeping together. At mine, never at his – that would be too risky, even for me. Strangely, I do not think of this as cheating, at least not in the true sense of the word. This is not – cannot be – cheating, not if it were meant to happen anyway. Who am I cheating? Not even myself.

This was always meant to happen, if not now then at some other point in the future. It's not even like I'm betraying Howie, I still love him but I *need* to be with Justin, how could I not? It would be like buying an ice-cream and letting it melt all over the floor; or getting on an empty train and not sitting down. Not sleeping with Justin wouldn't have made sense. If Howie understood then he'd understand why I need him so much. Justin cares so much about me. He seems to want what is best for me. The best of everything. He seems to know me so well.

"Take this; it'll make the shit stop." Justin pops a little white pill onto my tongue and rolls me onto my back where the flat inner surface of my arm is visible. I can he is toying with the idea of adding to that mutiny of tiny red pinpricks. But there are just too many to risk it. Veins are so delicate after-all. They are so fragile, like the nice doctor said, carry on like that and your veins are going to collapse. I need my veins to stay solid, I need them solid or I'll collapse too. I'll collapse and die, and I don't want to, not like this.

Lami Okrekson

We are at my house; Stella is not home so she can't accuse me of anything: fucking around with two men? They don't want the same things from me, so it doesn't really count. Isn't this just one man I have created?

While Justin has me here on my back we might as well have some of the sex we came here to have, which we do. Then we roll over onto our backs (or at least Justin does, I am already on mine) and light a couple of Marlboros. I light two at once and pass one over. "Why do people always smoke cigarettes after sex?" I ask Justin, because he knows all the answers. He doesn't know the answer to this one.

"What does it matter?" He asks back. "The box is red." I accept this as the most I'm going to get out of him, and smoke the rest of my cigarette in silence. After the cigarettes are smoked, Justin gets up to leave.

Now that he has gone, the house feels empty and silent. Since Stella isn't here – or Alice – I am all alone in this place. Strangely, as much as I hate Stella, she makes me feel safe. Like when she's here, the bad things can't happen. The bad men who lurk in the shadows in the attic wouldn't dare come down while a real adult was present. Not like me, some little eighteen year old who hasn't even learned how to drive.

I sit on my bed and start crying, for no reason at all except for the fact that I am actually alone. These are not the huge attention-seeking tears, these are real, silent tears meant for nobody

DRIPFEED

but me. As suddenly as the tears come, they stop. Crying drains me, always, makes me feel less than I am; empty and dead inside. But not lighter, heavier. The tears take away from me, but they also add – something I can't quite put my finger on, all I know is that it's heavy and cold and only comes when I am alone. It's so heavy that it's pinning me to the bed, where I am so drained I can't even move my head. This lethargy is not physical, it is purely emotional.

I lay on the bed for ages, not even bothering to move my arms when the pins and needle start.

Eventually, the pain in my left arm becomes too much to handle and I am forced to move out of this position. On the bedside table next to me are two boxes of my xyzal levocetirizine dihydrochloride antihistamine tablets. In a new burst of energy I take all the packets out and start popping the tiny white pills onto my bed sheets. I sift them through my fingers, enjoying the cool feel of them, and make pretty shapes on the sheets. Then I empty them into an empty bag I found on the floor – left over from Stewie's cocaine.

In total, I have about fifty pills. My back door in case of emergency. They make me feel secure, not because I want to die, but because I know that I'll always have that option. The chance to take that back door out if all the shit gets too much for me to handle again. I won't, but if I need to, I can take that little bag, a small bottle of something pure and distilled, and escape from this borrowed life. I can give it back before the contract runs out. Who cares anyway? It's all borrowed; borrowed time, borrowed lives. None of it belongs to us; it's all on loan until we make enough mistakes to pay it back. What if I want to make all my mistakes now and get it over with? Or, what if I just don't bother? What if I take that little, plastic bag and let go? No one said a contract had to be ridden out to the very end. In the case of *fly-or-die*, I'd rather die.

    I don't do anything with the pills of course; I just put them in my drawer of illegal-and-dangerous things. I do, however, wonder if those fifty pills would even be enough to do it. How many of them it would take. How long, between me popping the first pill and laying down on the hardwood, it would take for the little white dots to do their damage. Surely fifty Xyzal would kill me; surely Stella wouldn't even have enough time for the caring-mother skit. Surely I'd be dead before I hit the floor.

I lie back on the bed and light another Marlboro, all my energy has gone again. Empty, cold stuff back in my stomach.

DRIPFEED

Chapter 11

"What is wrong with you? What is so wrong with you now, that you have to walk around in this zombie-like state all the time?"

"You should be glad I'm not a whore," I say. "You should be glad I'm not *shaming* you in public. You should be glad that I'm only doing it in the privacy of my own room." Stella tries to stare me down for a moment; it doesn't work.

"And what *are* you doing in your room?" She asks. "*Drugs*? Planning your next overdose? What will it be this time *Chuck*," – she spits my name like she's choking on it – "more sleeping pills? Pain-killers? *Rat poison*? I wouldn't put it past you. You know, I sometimes wish I'd never had you."

"Why did you then?" I ask nonchalantly, not even offended by her insult. "You could have had an abortion, or you could have just kept your legs closed. I didn't ask to be born – like I said before, you brought me into this world, deal with it."

Stella sighs. "God knows I've tried." She says this looking up, as though God is actually agreeing with her.

This usual back and forth would have once left me so upset I'd have been right upstairs with the razor blades and the Valium, hacking away at my wrists and telling myself it was too unbearable to handle. Now that I have Justin, nothing could drive me to such extremes. Stella's insults don't phase me at all, they merely bore me; acting as an inconvenience, a distraction preventing me from doing anything else.

I catch grungy woman and Howie whispering in the kitchen. They instantly come apart when I enter, which is why I can't help thinking the word *caught* instead of *found*. The fact that they stopped talking when I entered makes me think they were talking about me. The problem with Chuck. What's new? What to do about me, with me; how *I* am creating this huge problem that *needs* to be solved. I have become a problem, like a leaky tap or a broken cistern; I need to be fixed by a repairman who knows how to fix *me.*

It doesn't occur to me that Howie and grungy-looking woman are doing anything other than talking. It doesn't occur to me that I might not be the only unfaithful one in this relationship. So I get my drink and go, leaving them – I think – to go on discussing me.

As I walk away from the door I hear peals of laughter, from the woman, and stifled giggle, from Howie. Now I know they are talking about me, what else could it be? The laughter continues as I move towards the living room and sit down. Even through all the music and chatter, I think I can still hear them. Someone offers me a joint, but I refuse.

Stella was right. Even *I've* noticed my zombie-like state. I occasionally find myself drooling – like

DRIPFEED

when I've done some spray paint – if I'm sitting still doing nothing. And often, I am not even thinking, just sitting, not even watching. This must be what meditation is like; clearing your mind of everything but the tiny little bell you're supposed to ring.

      Now I know what people mean when they say, drugs kill your brain cells; I can practically feel them dying one-by-one. When I wake in the morning I will be one less brain cell closer to the loony bin, the place where the inmates are so crazy they are licking the strawberry wallpaper off the walls, and hoarding supplies of laxatives. Just in case. In case of what? I'd ask. Just in case.

If we put as much effort into our education's as we do to our obsessions we'd be geniuses. Who knows, we may have even found a cure for AIDS and cancer by now. Perhaps. It's funny how closely related the word meditation is to medication.

I decide to do something, other than Howie or Justin, or the endless supply they dripfeed into me. I go to Leeds again, alone this time. It will give me a chance to have my first retrospective, or at least provide me with some kind of revelation. Since I'm travelling incognito this time, and have no car of my own, I am forced to Megabus it up here with about fifty other sweaty people. The journey is not difficult, aside from images of buses full of children crashing and colliding with trees. I manage to remain calm. I am not obliged to talk to the man sitting next to me; I don't even bother smiling at him when he sits down. I tried to repel him, with the evil eye that said, just keep walking bitch. But it didn't work; he sat his big, leather-jacket-wearing-in-the-summertime self down next to me.

I can't stand the smell of BO, and this man had it *bad*. I must have managed to block him out, because when we arrive at the Metro bus depot in Leeds four and a half hours later, I have no recollection of the journey. The fat man smiles at me – unreturned, of course – and I get off the bus, at a loss again. Fuck!

As I'm walking around this city that doesn't look so hot anymore now that I am experiencing it alone, Howie calls.

"Where are you?" He asks.

"Leeds."

"Leeds?"

"Yes," I say.

"What are you doing in Leeds?"

"I don't know." I am being truthful. I honestly do not know what I am doing in Leeds. What possessed me to book that one-way ticket, last minute so it wasn't even a pound anymore? I don't know what even made me think I had enough money to fund this little escapade. Howie is silent on the other end, probably wondering what to do about me again. I expect the grungy-looking woman is there on the other end, listening in on the speaker-phone, patting his shoulder, telling him not to worry, how brave he is to put up with all my shit.

DRIPFEED

"Why didn't you tell me?" He finally says.

"I didn't know until today."

"What do you mean, you 'didn't know until today?' How did you even get there?" He's probably thinking I hitched a ride with some drunken scumbag; probably thinks I'm off to live in a tree house with that same drunk scumbag. I almost pity him, then it dawns on me, he is treating me like a child, yet again. For fucks sake! In the eyes of the law, of Britain, I am a legal adult; I am more than capable of making my own decisions. I don't need anyone holding my hand every time I want to take a bus ride by myself. Why can't anyone understand that?

"I got the bus," I finally say, even though Howie doesn't actually have the right to ask me all these questions. He's hardly talking to me these days anyway. He's too busy talking *about* me to that fucking woman in the grey sweater. Still in the grey sweater! Weeks after I first saw her in it. She's a grown woman, if she doesn't have a washing machine, I'm sure she has enough twenty pence pieces to make use of a launderette. In fact, I don't even know why she's there. I come in and she's there, I wake up and she's there, I go to take a shit and she's there. All the fucking time. Always in my face, just like everyone else. Even the people walking past me on the road, wondering why this bitch is walking around in circles, can't help staring at me – like I'm wearing their underwear or something.

"You took the Megabus to Leeds? By yourself!" Howie's tone is incredulous, like I purposefully set out to hurt him. Like this was a premeditated attempt to attack him.

"Yeah, so what?"

"Anything could have happened."

"Like what?" I say. "What is going to happen to me, between me getting on and off of a bus that could be of any actual harm?"

"I didn't say inside the bus," Howie says. "Where are you even staying tonight? When were you planning on coming back? Did you even book a return ticket?" Questions! Too many questions.

"In that place we stayed in."

"With the rats and cockroaches? Do you even know where it is?"

"Oh for fucks sake Howie! Can't I do something by myself, without having you or Stella in my face? Why do you need to treat me like a child all the time? I was fine before you, remember, I had a life before you! What's so fucking different now that you have to be so protective all the time?"

"I'm just trying to be your friend," he says. "If I wasn't so concerned you'd probably be angry with me for not caring. Now that I am caring, you think it's too much. I don't know how to *be* with you, without you going all psycho bitch all the time."

"*I'm* going psycho bitch?" I say. "What about you? Who phoned who here? I didn't phone you asking you millions of questions. I didn't even ask you to phone me. *You* decided to. I just wanted to take a little break!"

DRIPFEED

"You should have just said. I would have come with you."

"Howie, you don't get it. I wanted to be alone; I need some time to sort out the shit in my head. You all want me gone anyway, so here I am."

"Why is it always about you?" Howie asks.

"You *made* it about me when you called!" It's silent on the other end and I think that Howie has hung up. Although if *I* had hung up on him, I would have slammed the receiver down so he could hear it, I wouldn't have silently accepted defeat. Howie isn't violent enough for that. He's too soft to do anything other than raise his voice and put the phone down gently. Quietly blocking me out with his fingers in his ears.

"I called because I wanted you to come out tonight. We're going to see this band play."

"Oh…why didn't you just say?" I feel stupid for making this into a big drama. I'll leave here without the retrospective, *or* the revelation. All I will have succeeded in doing is wasting yet more of the money I don't have, and driving another wedge between Howie and me.

"Because." And I don't even need to say, because what? Because I know. It's because I shouldn't be here in Leeds anyway. This is not something even *I* was expected to do. "Do you need me to come and pick you up?" Howie asks.

Yes! Yes I do need you to come and pick me up. I need a ride; I need to be told what an idiot I am. Maybe it will make me see what everyone else sees when they look at me. A wasted youth. A girl still clinging onto those childhood illusions long after everyone else has left the party. "No. I'll find my own way back," I reply. "I'll find an internet café or something, and book a bus today."

"You won't find one."

"Then I'll stay." Howie must have said, fine, but I can't be sure. All I know is the line goes dead, and when I look at my phone, the call has ended. I end up spending another night in a cheap bed 'n' breakfast. This one is as shitty and as cockroach-infested-looking as the other one. I spend the entire night lying on the lumpy bed with the lights on. This time I am not taking any chances. Those cockroaches are not going to get the chance to come crawling all over me again.

When I get back to London the next day, I go straight to Howie's flat – unashamed, un-showered, un-brushed. He isn't talking to me again, nothing new there. I can't find Justin so I just go home. Stella isn't there either, I didn't tell her I was going out, on account of the fact that I didn't know. I expected some sort of welcome-home party though, that is Stella dragging me in by the face, demanding – always demanding – to know where I've been, with whom, what time I call it, the usual. But she isn't here, Alice isn't here. The house is as vacant and silent as when I left it. Nothing has changed, no one missed me, no one even knew I was gone.

The same dishes from yesterday are still in the sink, the same unopened letters are still on the

DRIPFEED

table. I went away, came back, and nothing had changed. I might as well have stayed. If anything, things got worse: Howie's giving me the silent treatment, if Stella found out I was gone she'll have her knife in me as well. I might as well get my own knife and save them all the trouble.

I take my bag upstairs and drop it on the floor. My room looks different, bare like a hotel. I take a cigarette out of the packet and light up. I feel like a guest here.

Chapter 12

I don't know what to do; yesterday I spent another night at Howie's. After listening to yet more musical debates we went into Howie's bedroom and lay down on the bed. We didn't do anything except smoke a few cigarettes and exchange a few monosyllabic words. We went to sleep thinking of that yucky after-taste cigarette smoke leaves in your mouth.

I am standing on my rug deciding what to wear today. It doesn't matter, I'll probably spend the whole day trying to figure out how I'm going to haul all my stuff up to university anyway – since Howie is out of the question and I don't want to bother with Stella. There is just so much stuff, too much stuff, most of it junk that I can't be bothered to throw away: old primary school paintings, clay sculptures, text books, clothes and shoes I never wear anymore, and so many CD's. So many that it would probably take an entire army months just to get through all the intros. It occurs to me that one car may not be enough for all the stuff I have accumulated over the years. I'll end up as the only undergraduate to turn up with a removal van.

I can't decide what to wear so I just go back to bed. When I wake up Justin is beside me. He must have been there when I first got up, though I can't remember. There is just so much emptiness inside my head. I can't even remember if I was alone before I fell asleep.

DRIPFEED

That's when the voices start coming back. The weird, niggling voices in the back of my head. The ones telling me I'm shit, that I'm less than shit, not even worthy of this crack head, junky beside me. That I'm not worthy of the air I'm breathing, the body I'm borrowing, that I'm just plain unworthy; like the Un-women from *A Handmaids Tale*. I should be banished to some toxic waste land to die pointlessly sweeping toxic debris into neat little piles. The return of these voices doesn't surprise me at all. When I tell Justin about them he tells me to shush, and injects, rolls, inhales, blows. If I told Howie, he would sigh and roll over to face the wall, or prepare to leave me again like everyone else did.

Justin never became fruitful like Howie, who was so fucking quiet in the beginning of this thing we have, so unwilling to volunteer anything other than his time and his stash. Justin never says anything except for, I know what you want, or, you want this don't you? It seems that Howie, like Ezra, really has had it with the class A's. Along with grungy-looking woman, all I ever see him do is weed – and that doesn't really count anyway, since it's practically legal now. He sighs and runs a hand through his hair now, when he sees the inside of my arms. You can't keep doing this, he says. You're gonna make yourself really ill if you do. He doesn't cry anymore, when he says this.

Justin and I continue to do what we do, although we do it less because I need to spend more time alone, looking into the water, fighting the urges to jump in, trying to spot one of the fish that are supposed to be in there, or a stray shark that made its way here from the sea, or the ocean if it was feeling adventurous enough. I do these things all by myself, without chaperoning from Howie or Chavez or Justin. I spend so much time up here on the bridge because I am avoiding Starbucks. The one-nighter called me. And called me and called me. I'm too scared to even walk past a Starbucks now, who knows what they do in there, if they ship them around like salesmen, from shop to shop, branch to branch.

Strange as it may seem, I have no use for him now. I just wanted the release that his body gave me. No one said he had to be so fucking clingy. *I'm* supposed to be the clingy one, not them. Not Howie, or Chavez, or Justin, or the ones who didn't bother calling.

The first thing Justin does when I wake him up is to reach into his jeans pocket and take out two pills, one of which he slips into my mouth, and the other into his. I swallow obediently, I don't even know what this shit is. We are all just a gang of losers I suppose, listening to Radiohead in our time off, depressing ourselves voluntarily. We love self-destruction, why wouldn't we? We are a nation of sado-masochists, self-mutilation is our forté.

DRIPFEED

The pill starts working, it must have been ecstasy because I feel - contrary to Ezra's little anecdote, like a butterfly that has just been released from its cocoon. I want to dance. Correction. I want to dance like no one's watching in front of everyone. This feeling of elation only lasts a few moments of course, because seconds later I'm chewing the inside of my face like it's a hot wing from KFC. Then I start burning. Burning and chewing my face all in the same motion. I try clenching my jaw, but that just makes it worse. My mind goes back to these dreams I used to have, about my jaw locking and all my teeth snapping off. I know this is what's happening. My dream was some weird kind of premonition, and now it's coming true. I'm going to sit here on the bed chewing my face to a bloody pulp while all my teeth snap and crackle out of my head. I look over at Justin, who is remarkably fine. He went back to sleep, apparently this shit doesn't affect him like it affects me.

I'm so hot I feel like I've got the flu. I wish there was some kind of lake out there, something that I could just jump into to cool all this burning shit off. I want to sleep. I can't. I'm so uncomfortable and hot that I can't even focus on the foam squares on the ceiling. There is just too much shit going on in my head - that and the fact that my lower jaw is now somewhere in the vicinity of my shoulder - that I would gladly accept the blankness I had before the voices started infiltrating again.

Eventually I go and sit in the bathroom, without getting in the tub, just looking at the white enamel, imagining slipping beneath ice cold water. It is enough to cool the burning across my skin, and gradually my jaw eases itself back into a position I can handle.

While I'm in here cooling down, I take out my phone and call Chavez. I didn't plan on calling her; in fact I haven't spoken to her in ages. It's late, or early, and she isn't answering. I am persistent though, without Ezra I have no one else to be my psychiatrist. I thought my demons couldn't be fed and pulled out with incessant chatter. Bullcrap! All that fucking shit just to make other people feel better. I thought I didn't have the time to waste. That was bullshit. Ezra was my rock for so long that without him I need Ezra-replacements. The real Ezra is too busy for me now, with his styling and his shopping, so I *have* to find the replacement Ezras: Belle, Howie, Chavez, Justin. It all amounts to the same thing, these people are just my coping mechanisms, my tooth fairies and Easter bunnies, things I need to take the edge off and come to grips with the fact that yes! I am alone.

I could always go to Ezra's, even though he isn't there. His parents would welcome me with open arms. This makes me cry how these people would invite me into their home without a second thought and fill my head with more philosophical bullshit than I can handle.

DRIPFEED

I am crying when Chavez finally answers the phone. "Chuck!" She says. "Long time baby." I am crying so hard now that I can't even speak. She is not used to this side of me, apart from the little incident in the wardrobe; she thinks I'm just as fucked up as she is. Some other self-destructive teenager on a mission to get high. A young junky with nothing better to do than see how long my veins will last before they completely collapse. "What's wrong Puss?" She asks. We're about ten minutes into this conversation and here I am still crying over nothing more than the fact that my best friend's parents like me. Shit! "Want me to come over to yours?" I'm not even making any attempt to stop this Niagara Falls shit in my tear ducts. "Chuckie baby, are you there?"

"Yes," I finally manage after quickly putting this thing into perspective and realising that I am indeed being a tad stupid. Finally!

"So what's up?"

"Nothing." Nothing is up as usual. I just wanted someone else to share the dark with me.

"I haven't seen you in ages," I say. "Did I wake you up?"

"Nah. I don't sleep at night. You know that."

"Yeah." Silence. This is not unusual for a phone conversation between Chavez and me. We have nothing to say to each other.

"What's the matter?" She asks.

"I'm under construction." I say. "I need time to calm the voices in my head."

Lami Okrekson

"We've all got voices in our heads." This is what I like about Chavez, the fact that where anyone else would have said, 'I think you should talk to someone,' Chavez just lets me be crazy. "Sure you don't want me to come over?" She sounds bored, like she couldn't give a shit what I want her to do, as long as she can get off this phone and away from the monotony that has been my life for the past few months.

"Yeah, I'm sure."

"Okay then. Well I'm gonna go, things to do baby. We'll hook up soon though."

???????????????

I am Chuck. I am scared of ceiling fans and I am flakier than a 99p flake from Mr. Whippy's. Sorry. I'll let you down but I'll make it up to you later. I can't help it, it's who I am. I am also a coward. I hate your shoes but I'll tell you I love them. I tell more lies than Anton LeVay but I'm not a Satanist. I talk in riddles and no one gets what I mean. All the rumours you heard about me were probably true. I am not as elusive as I may seem.

After the phone conversation with Chavez I feel cool enough not to burn between the sheets. I go back into my bedroom and lie down on my bed. I stare at my foam ceiling, glad that there are no moths or cockroaches up there. I fall asleep looking at my clock, counting sheep and trying to keep Justin from hitting me in the face in his sleep.

DRIPFEED

When I wake up again I am alone. No Justin, no weird ecstasy burning me up from the inside. No Chavez telling me she has to go. Just me. Now, in the light of day, I wonder if all that really happened, or if I just dreamt it up in my crazy imagination. Perhaps this is what they meant when they said drugs fry your brain. Maybe my brain is so fried that I can't remember if I dreamt Justin in my bed, or if he was really there. There is nothing in my room to suggest anyone other than me was here. No sock on the floor, Calvins rolled in a ball under the bed, not even the faint after-scent of sex and after-shave lingering in the air. I lay back on my bed, I might as well, I am clearly too insane to do anything else.

We are the ones who fill your head with so much crap you don't know whether to thank us with a million dollar tip or throw us over the side of an ocean liner. Your only problem with us is that we don't care enough to piss you off, and that pisses you off. We took everything you gave and didn't even say thank you.

I'm back in Howie's bed, with Howie, smoking a Marlboro under some giant invisible question mark. The story of my life and all the pages are blank; like the *Never Ending Story*. If we had the choice to be born, knowing all this shit - all the arse fucking and expletives at the beginning of every sentence - who'd choose it? Answer; no one would. We would tie our umbilical chords around our partially developed necks and choke ourselves to death.

We walk through Carnaby street - Howie and I - underneath the sign that says '*WELCOME TO CARNABY STREET*', even though we are clearly leaving it; like the signs that say '*Welcome to Greenwich*', when you are clearly entering Lewisham. I decided to get those Vans after all, since Howie offered to foot the bill. So here we are, walking away from Carnaby Street, towards Regent Street where Howie can look in the windows of all the shops he likes and tell himself that he too will one day be affluent enough to buy more than a pair of socks from any one of those oh-so-pretentious retail outlets. Howie and I hold hands. For a moment we remind me of a real couple.

Back at home, trying on the Vans, realising that I don't like them so much - now that they're off the display and on my feet. Throw them to the back of the wardrobe with all the other shit I buy and then don't wear.

    I will never wear those shoes again, all those black and white squares, all this chequered shit is just too attention-grabbing, at a time I wish to remain so elusive; like Banksy or Gnarls Barkley. All this is just more stuff I'll have to take to university. All of it just means bigger suitcases, more suitcases, a bigger van even, maybe two. Why can't I just throw shit away and be done with it like everyone else? Why is stuff always so much easier to do in theory? In practice it's just too hard.

The date book on my phone puts today at the sixth of September. Alice started school today, a year up, matured by the summer - just like everything else, except for me.

How could so much time have passed so quickly when it seemed to be going so slowly at the time? Three months. Three short months since I met Chavez, decided class A's were better than orange juice, and became a self-confessed junky. I can hardly believe this ride is almost over already, that in a few weeks I'll be packing to move on again. I'll be locked inside another institution for another three years. It's funny how things always come in threes.

Justin and I hardly ever see each other anymore. He was bad for me, worse than Chavez, worse than any dealer I've ever encountered. He was worse because he made me believe he was good for me, he made me believe he was doing me a favour by fucking my life up like he did. And anyway, he was getting bored. He would have ended things if I hadn't.

It took me so long to see through Justin. Three weeks, to be exact, to see exactly what he was doing, how much he enjoyed seeing me too strung out to remember my own name. He got a kick out of watching me fall over every time I tried to get up. And stupid me didn't even realise until right at the end when he was getting fed up with me anyway.

We had just arrived at his, having spent the last few hours devouring my stash, when he practically shot a spliff into my hand. I knew I had done way too much, in fact I felt like I was bordering on "overdose" again. Familiar feelings of my brain being a tad *too* chilled out. I was not in the zone at that point, I was way outside of it, on the other side of sanity - too far away from okay to be okay, let alone do any more of that.

For the first time in my career as a "yes" person I pushed it away. I behaved like the good little Catholic girl Stella brought me up to be, and said NO! Then it clocked in my head, that Justin hardly ever did as much shit as I did. He was always the one to shoot me up, to light a spliff, take one pull and then pass it along to me. We never fucked sober, or at least I was always too fucked to say no, or even want to say no. It was always Justin handing me the bag saying, you want this don't you? Always him pressing those tiny white pills onto the tip of my tongue and going back to sleep. How could I have been so stupid? Love is blind, not lust.

In fact, the day I said no was the only time I'd seen Justin do coke. He did it right in front of me, emptied the bag onto the table and inhaled as if to entice me. I could not be enticed. Weak as I am, I retained some form of dignity and looked away.

DRIPFEED

Howie walked in, frowning at the coke, assuming that I was the one who initiated it, looking at me like I was betraying him, even though I never said I would quit too. I couldn't stand to be around either of them, so I went home and drowned my sorrows in a little bottle of Jack Daniels. Little enough that I could afford it, large enough to get me smashed enough to fall asleep and forget about it.

Chapter 13

Alice got some experiment to do at school, one of those ones where you put things in a bowl of water and note down which of them sinks and which of them swims. I don't know why they gave this experiment to Alice; she knows what sinks and what doesn't. They should have known they were dealing with a mini-genius the minute she walked in. She would have been the only one whose tie was exactly one metre long, tucked into a perfectly ironed shirt, every book weighing down that enormous backpack. They would have never believed we came from the same vagina.

Stella came bursting into my room brandishing an empty Jack Daniels bottle. "What is this?"
"Duh. What does it look like? It's not fucking Coca Cola, is it?" Alice had it. She was using it in her 'sink or swim' experiment. There Stella goes, thinking I'm going to turn her precious baby into a junky like me, or worse, an alcoholic like her.
"When did you start drinking whisky? She demands.
"When did I start drinking whisky?" I repeat. "How about asking when I started popping sleeping pills with vodka, or waking up in cupboards with knives in my arms."
"I don't understand you, Charlotte."
"That's okay, no one does. You're not the only one who doesn't understand me. I'm elusive."

DRIPFEED

"Why can't you speak like a normal human being for once?" She asks. "Why must you go round and round with these riddles all the time?"

"They're not riddles," I spit at her. "You just don't understand my English. You said so yourself."

She changes the subject here, because she knows I'm right - as always. And I am always right when it comes to her. "You had to involve your sister didn't you? You just had to drag Alice into your self-destructive little world."

"I didn't drag Alice anywhere," I defend. Why the fuck is she always pulling me off as the bad one? "She found an empty bottle in my room. She used it in a science experiment. She didn't drink it."

Stella gives one of her legendary sighs. "I don't know why you have to disappoint me so much." She says this quietly, under her breath almost, a telltale sign her own Niagara Falls is about to start. Any minute now she's going to break down into gelatine - so I'll feel sorry for her no doubt.

"*You* disappoint *me*," I say. "So we're even-fucking-Stevens, aren't we?"

Stella comes further into the room, looking with disgust at the clothes all over the floor, the cigarette butts deposited in various ash trays across the wood, her nostrils flare; she doesn't like the smell of incense. "Why don't you just leave?" She says, so matter-of-factly that it takes me a while to fully understand the sarcasm underneath the question. "Go. If you want to. You do want to, don't you? Take your incense and your cigarettes and get out. I don't pay the bills so you can come in here and fuck things up with your smoke and your candles. You're an adult, you're eighteen, and you're old enough to look after yourself. You don't need me, do you? I don't look after you; I'm just here to make your life miserable - that's what you think, isn't it?"

She leaves the room and comes back with a suitcase. She starts grabbing things off the floor and shoving them into the suitcase. "Here, I'll help you," she says. "You want to leave and I'm not going to stop you. Take your - clothes, and your shoes..." she throws more things into the case. "...and go. I want you out of here!" She throws the half-packed case onto the floor, scattering a few cigarette butts out of their ash trays and onto *her* hardwood, then she leaves again. I sit there for a while before lighting a cigarette and dragging the smoke deep into my lungs. Smoking kills! It says so on the packet. Fuck it. Stella bursts back in, "You treat this place like a hotel, coming and going as you please. Smoking! Leaving all this shit on the floor for me to clean up."

"But you don't, do you?" I spit. "You don't clean my shit up because you don't care."

"You're right," she agrees. "I don't care." She leaves again and I light another cigarette with the half-smoked one in my hand.

I wish there was something I could take to erase her from my life for good. I want to hurt her more than she's ever hurt me - the Stella-proof vest isn't

DRIPFEED

working anymore. I want to freeze the moment her heart breaks and then replay it over and over again. I want to smash her heart on the floor and trample on it, except I wouldn't cut my feet because I would be immune to her and her heart and her blood and anything else remotely connected to her.

There is though, no way I can think of, nothing I could do to hurt her even as much as she's hurt me. The only way I can truly get back at her is if I kill myself. If I shoot myself in the head on top of a car in the middle of the street. If everybody was standing outside, open-mouthed, shivering in their cotton dressing gowns, checking upstairs windows to make sure the kids were still asleep, trying not to stare but not even pretending anymore. I'd be like a fucking train wreck. They couldn't look away if their lives depended on it.

The suicide wouldn't be the thing that broke her though, I don't mean enough to her for that. It'd be the sheer humiliation, the laying bare of her soul in front of people - people she never even bothered to say 'good morning' to. I am her fucking heart attack, and every minute I course through he veins is the best fucking minute of my life. It's not the fact that she is ruining my life that is not the problem, life is irrelevant, it isn't even guaranteed. Life is like waiting for the bus, or an orgasm while eating potato salad. It's just something to do in between the toe-tapping and tail-gating. If I had the choice between life and watching her break, I'd throw life to the fishes in the river Thames. Who needs it? It's a bitch and all that, can't help fucking you in the arse when you've just about been fucked by everything else: school, exams, money, no money, boys, men, no boys, too many men. And Stella is the baddest of the bad. Bad people like her don't even deserve to go to hell. The only punishment suitable for such a mark on society is to be broken. To be so incredibly broken that you can't even remember what your life looked like as one entity. All you have left are the tiny shards of shattered shit messing up the hardwood.

After I smoked the second cigarette I lit some more incense sticks and waved them around in the air a bit. I brushed my teeth to get rid of that smoky taste I hate, and took an aspirin for my psychosomatic headache. Then I drank flat cherry Tango straight out of the bottle. I did all this without realising. But not mechanical like a robot, more robotic like a machine. I must have come face-to-face with her then. I don't remember. I probably don't even register her existence anymore. Fucking cunt! She doesn't exist in my world of heroin and cucumber sandwiches.

    I gave myself a hit on the bathroom floor and somehow made it back to my room, choking on pungent air. I forgot how to open windows long before I learned how to take a hit. And they said secondary school taught us nothing.

DRIPFEED

Chapter 14

It didn't surprise me one little bit that Justin never called; since he never did when we had our little thing anyway. Another transparent clue I should have seen straight through. I was always the one to call him. It was always me checking to see if the coast was clear - if Howie was out. It was always me saying, Stella's passed out again, come over. So when we finished it, I wasn't even expecting a text message. Of course I still went over there to see Howie. Surprisingly we are still together, despite grungy-looking woman, in spite of Justin.

My orange alarm clock wakes me up at the same time my phone rings. It's Howie. Who else would it be? No one bothers to call me these days.

"Do you wanna come over today?" He asks.

"What time?"

"Whenever." We have a brief conversation, like the ones in the beginning, punctuated with long, uncomfortable silences. Then we hang up and I get up like I intended.

It is well after ten and Alice is long gone, probably in a classroom somewhere arranging her stationary into neat little rows on her desk. Or, knowing the answers to the questions but not volunteering, her intelligence outweighed by her shyness. If only Stella had been a bit more encouraging. Courage. If only Stella had given us a bit more courage. Then what?

Lami Okrekson

I eat breakfast - alone in the kitchen because Stella is out, and I wouldn't be in there anyway if she were in there. We do not get along. Toast because I don't like Rice Krispies and Rice Krispies is all Stella ever buys. She knows I don't like them but she thinks Alice does. I happen to know that Alice would prefer Corn Flakes once in a while, or Cheerios - all that wholegrain goodness in those little, tiny O's. And they taste good to boot. Why wouldn't any normal eleven year old want them?

Back upstairs I think about what I'll wear today, not because I care but because I'm running out of clean clothes. Stella took the fuse out of the washing machine, probably to teach me a lesson. It bugs me because I need to wash my clothes and I am from a generation that has come to rely and depend upon modern electrical appliances. Other than that she can get on with whatever rocks her boat. She can ride this revenge tragedy out to the end. Pissed off because I came along and fucked everything up for her. Or because I'm not the straight 'A' student I used to be. Instead I'm the idiot who lost her GCSE results and had to pay for replacements.

Fucking bitch. Whatever makes her happy.

The only two things in my wardrobe that are clean aren't even that clean. I wear them anyway, since I have nothing else. Since Stella fucked that part of my life up too.

DRIPFEED

I take the long way to Howie's, getting off the tube at Waterloo so I can look in the water and throw all my troubles in there. The day care centre for the troubled mind, this place has become. I'll collect my shit when I come back here. I'll always come back here. How could I not?

The first thing I wonder when I step over Howie's threshold is what the fuck! Why would he invite me here at a time when there is so much temptation? So much for me to put into my body, so much shit to float into my bloodstream, so much junk to inhale. I haven't had my daily bread yet, my daily hit up the nasal passage, and I rub the side of my nose, prematurely feeling the pepper-like sting as that good shit hits my brain direct. The nose is the only direct route to the brain, i.e. coke up the nose fucks you up quicker.

The usual suspects are here as usual. The twenty or so people gathered around on chairs, in groups by the window, on the stairs. The air in here is thick with smoke and incense - Howie 'borrowed' a couple of sticks from me earlier in the week. Justin is here too, as always, lounging on the couch, wearing shades, smoking a joint while some hot, half-naked chick prepares to shoot heroin into his exposed inner arm. I can't believe Justin is smart enough to have orchestrated this for my benefit, to spite me. He didn't care about me enough to waste his time with stupid mind-games. Howie leads me to the sofa opposite

Justin and hands me a joint - dope is allowed, it's the class A's he has a problem with.

We smoke the joint and everything becomes soft around the edges. The people don't seem so harsh and jarring like they did before, even the air is starting to feel nice and cool against my skin. The feelings don't last long though. When it wears off I look around and all I see is a group of stoned teenagers and stoned men, getting drunk and swaying to death metal. Getting stoned with them does not seem like a good idea anymore.

I get up and find my way to the bathroom, where Justin is taking a piss - what do I care, I've seen it all before? I slump down on the floor with my back against the bath. This is an invitation and we both know it. Justin pulls a needle from his majestic stash and joins me on the floor, where he takes my arm and administers the shot.

I pass out for a bit and come too alone.

Justin left me a bag of which I devour. Then Howie comes in, again, with Justin in tow. "What the fuck!" he exclaims, running over to catch my head before it hits the floor. "What the fuck are you doing? I thought you said you were going to stop with this stuff. What are you doing?"

"Justin said it was okay," I say. Howie shoots Justin a look. Justin shrugs and lights another cigarette.

DRIPFEED

After carrying me into his bedroom and depositing me on the bed amid a pile of coats, Howie turns to me. We are alone now, no Justin with his Ray Bans smoking his weed by the door. Just us.

Even through the closed door, the party is still going strong. Muffled sounds and smells still creep through the crack at the bottom of the door. Music, laughter, a bottle dropping but not breaking on the beaten-up carpet. More laughter.

"I can't do this anymore," Howie is saying. "*You* can't keep doing this. Every time I think we're okay you go and pull a stunt like this. It's like you're trying to push me away. I loved you, you know." Loved? "Why do you keep doing this, Chuck? Part of me thinks you *were* trying to kill yourself that time. Part of me thinks you still are." I feel giddy from all the heroin and weed and cocaine. All the fumes from the party - the perfume and the incense, the smoke - filter into my brain, pure and distilled from under the door. These things make me laugh. "You're not even listening, are you?" Howie continues. "You don't even know what I'm saying. What happened to you? It was cool before; when you drank too much and passed out it was cute. Now it's just boring. What the fuck happened to you?" I'm still laughing a bit and Howie gets up and slams the door. Then he slams another door in another room. I stay on the bed for a while, listening to the party still going strong on the other side of the door. Then I get up and follow Howie across the hall to Stewie's room.

Lami Okrekson

I don't know what I expected to see when I opened the door. Or, if I did expect that, that it would hurt me as much as it did. I thought *I* cheated on him so I won't care if he cheats on me. I didn't know I really loved him too.

Howie is in there, in Stewie's bed, making love to grungy-looking girl. I say 'making love,' because that is exactly what it looks like from where I'm standing. They are not fucking or screwing, not like me and Justin. In some ways this love-making is worse than if I caught him fucking her. If he were just acting on impulse and not - as cliché as it may sound - from his heart, then maybe it wouldn't be so bad. Grungy-looking girl sees me standing there and gives me this smug, satisfied look. And there's nothing I can do about it; she knows it too. I stole her man before she stole mine. At least he loves her. I shut the door quietly, go find Justin, and lead him back to Howie's room. Two can play at that game, even though I have already played.

Justin and I do some lines, equal amounts this time - now that we have become equals. We take our clothes off but find we are too stoned to anything other than stare at yet another foam ceiling. There are two moths dangling from it, which makes me shudder. It makes Justin laugh. We lie like that for a while, side-by-side, bare skin barely touching. We don't talk; we have nothing left to say. Justin was my back up, my dick in a glass case - to break open in case of emergency. Now he's just the man who can. Bringing me

DRIPFEED

whatever poison I desire: animal, vegetable or mineral.

Howie comes back in from his love-making, to apologise no doubt. To tell me how sorry he was that we can work through this if I stop with the bullshit, that I'm not how I was before…blah blah fucking blah. Drugs schmugs. It's all the same to me. Whatever gets me high. More to the point, whatever gets me high *quickest.*

    He comes in and finds me and Justin in bed together, drags Justin out of the bed and punches him in the face. Kicks him out the door - the music gets louder for a second - turns to me. "Did you love him?" he spits - his voice is full of anger and venom I note, why? "Cos I loved you!"

    "Really?" I say. "Is that why you were in there fucking grungy-looking girl?"

    "Grungy-looking girl?" He is confused. "Oh. You mean Freya."

    Freya!

    "Whatever. You did, I did, so we're even Stevens, aren't we?"

    Howie looks upset for a moment, then nonchalant, then angry. "No we're not," he says quietly. "All those times I caught you over here. I thought you were just getting high."

    "And what about you?" I'm shouting, angry now at the irony of all this. "How long was it before you fucked her? Before or after she comforted you? Before or after I OD'd?"

    "Because of me."

"I told you, it was an accident." We both stand there for a moment, both in the wrong but neither bothering to acknowledge or admit it.

"Well we're obviously over," he finally says.

"Did *you* love *her*?" I have to know.

"Did *you* love *him*?"

"No."

Silence.

"Well?" I prompt.

"She listened to me. She didn't get high and do stupid things like…"

"Like me," I finish. "I take it you did, love her I mean."

"What does it matter?" He says. "We were over ages ago." It stings to hear this, even though I know it's true. I always thought we'd work it out, even after Justin and Starbucks guy. Even after Freya and Justin again. I thought we'd be okay. *We were over ages ago.* That means they've been going on longer than me and Justin. If I felt guilty about Starbucks guy before, I wouldn't now. Howie practically slapped me in the face with that. Even a slap would have been more forgivable.

How could I have been so stupid? How could I not have seen this? All those secretive conversations, peals of laughter erupting from behind closed doors. It was all about me. Always about me. Me. The *I am*. And I am me. And it wasn't. This time it was about them; them and their sordid little affair. Me again. There I go, pointing the finger when I fucked around too. Only after, so it doesn't really count.

DRIPFEED

I wanted to live in the fairytale. All I had to do was get there and it would have been okay. There in the place of golden bunnies with chocolate smiles that give everything away. I wanted it and I wanted it bad. Wanted to meet the person who rang my bell and ran away. Now I'm here, where it's all been fucked up again. Her. *Freya.* Freya-fucking-grunge. She took him, and all they left me with was a mouth full of pips. I can't believe I could have been so blind. So fucking blinded by nothing but lights. Sparks, electricity, that's all it was. Not love. Why? Me! Wake up and smell the bacon! Why the bacon? Why not the formaldehyde, or the pain of your soul cracking in a million tiny pieces of nothingness?
 WE ARE BLINDED BY LOVE!
 Who am I again? Because I really don't know anymore. It feels like if I looked in the mirror I'd be able to recognise myself. Except I do, and then I don't. Shit. This is the conspiracy theory they were talking about. It has to be. They tag us; drain all our blood, and then we forget who we are.

For once I leave before he has the chance to. I go home and lay on the floor listening to Radiohead through stereo speakers. This pain is too great to be drowned out through headphones. I stay there, straight-laced and ignoring the pains of withdrawal.
 I could quit if I wanted to.

Chapter 15

Addicted. I try that word out in my head, add the prefix 'I am,' make a new sentence. Am I, or am I? I *am* addicted. No fronting this time. No pretending I'm not when I clearly am. I have now become dependant. Now? Or then? When? I so should have seen this coming. Aren't I the one always proclaiming the predictability of the human race? I am a part of that endless trap of cold spaghetti, and I couldn't even predict myself away from it.

I felt them, not for the first time, the pains of withdrawal. That's how I knew I'd know. When those pains hit. Cramps worse than period pains, cold sweats after a day. Maybe that's why they call it cold turkey; a frozen turkey still needs to be thawed after all.

The problem is simple this time. This time it is simply me. In fact I *did* see this coming - my one claim to fame being foresight, I knew this is where I'd end up eventually. Everyone else managed to get out before the train crashed. I decided to stay on. How can I possibly pull my mangled body from the wreckage alone? I can't. I'll lie here until I die, or until it wears off. I have no choice but to lie, it hurts less this way.

Why is it always me? Why am I always the one who gets too caught up in the moment and decides to stay on with a bunch of strangers? I should have known then. This hindsight bullshit is

DRIPFEED

just another kick up the arse, another ironic slap in the face - well ha ha and better luck next time!

And it's like, so many decisions, so many decisions and not enough time. Not enough space in my head for all these decisions. I want to go blank, break down, hysterical amnesia. I want to forget about the past few months. Go back to when it started getting increasingly shitter. Pause, rewind. Start all over again. Anew this time. No scars, no scar tissue; just me.

But I am addicted.

I am trapped in this downward spiral to the bottom of the well and the motion is making me sick. It's funny, that I am my own motion sickness, but I am also the cure. I wish I knew how to stop this thing. No one ever told us that, how to stop. They taught us how to avoid, defer, deflect. Stay away and don't even look! One look was all it took after all, before it dragged me in. But there's nothing about getting out. All those books on how to say 'no' to peer pressure, and not one about pulling your head out of the freezer. I just want it to stop. I want this to be over so I can carry on. I'll need more of that then, thank you.

I've still got the lighter. The one I got from the tattoo shop in Camden. The one I've been using religiously throughout this train ride. Neon pink when pink is so not my colour. The gas is running out. If I hold it up to the light I can see how much I have left. If. But the lights are never on and the curtains are always closed.

I light a spliff I must have rolled earlier, careful not to use too much gas. I smoke the spliff, but it's not enough. Not even to distract me for a while. Truthfully, I hardly feel it. I might as well be smoking a cigarette for all the good it does. I lie back feeling worse. That was just more smoke to add to an already smoky mind. I want to be clear. I need to think clearly again, and I can't, not without it. Without that thing that I was so scared of in the beginning. The thing that feels so good. The snake bite that releases such intoxicating venom I feel it for days.

I need those little blue men now, the ones with all that strawberry flavoured Vicodin. I can't carry on in this borrowed skin without them. It's enough to reduce me to tears, but I've just about cried myself dry over the last few months. There isn't even a reserve, a 'just-in-case-of,' I'm bone dry at a time when all I want to do is weep. And it's cold, so cold. But I can't take my head out of the freezer. I need it! Now!

!!!!!!!!!!!!!!!!!!!!!!!!!

DRIPFEED

Chapter 16

I call Chavez. She comes prepared. "Want me to shoot you up, Puss?" she says at the door. She puts the needle to my vein, draws blood and then pumps the bloody mixture back into my arm. A feeling like no other grips me from the abdomen and spreads like a thousand hands massaging me into a beautiful numbness. This is perfection.

We spend days under my duvet, watching Jeremy Kyle and eating popcorn chicken from KFC, shooting each other up on breaks. Snorting coke when we run out of heroin. Sniffing spray paint when we run out of coke. Listening to Radiohead when the paint runs dry.

Over these days, the popcorn chicken and the under-my-duvet drug sessions, it does not dawn on me that my relationship is actually over and I have no one again.

The mayfly only lives for one day.

After Chavez leaves - she starts school earlier than me - I call Howie. And I call him and I call him. He doesn't pick up. All I get is his voicemail. So I try Justin instead. "Fuck off!" He says when he finally picks up. So even Justin's deserted me. The only one who would be there under any circumstances, no matter what. He fucked and ran too.

Lami Okrekson

When I get off the phone with Justin I lie on the floor and concentrate on what to do next. I did not expect this ache. It seems too distant, too alien, to be real. I could call Chavez again, drag her away from her degree, get her over here to shoot me up and laugh at the Chavs on Jeremy Kyle. Or Ezra even, drag him away from his Miss Selfridge to dry my tears, listen to me rant about suicide and depression, the very things that drove him away in the first place. I could always go over to Howie's, bang on the door, or storm in - I still have the key - demand that we sort this out. Get down on my knees and weep and beg, while *Freya* shoots me poisonous looks from her place in Howie's heart.

Or I could end it. My answer to everything - why bother when it's all shit anyway?

I slit my wrists again.

There is a knife on the floor under the rug, always there just in case I need it. I need it now, don't I? I bring the knife to my wrist and tease the skin with its point. Dragging across, but not deep enough to draw blood. It scratches the skin, leaving white marks, and it feels good. Then I press deeply and slice the motherfucker open. The thing is it isn't my hand doing it. It feels like someone else's hand is drawing the knife across my veins, so sharp that all I can feel is the blood spilling hot across my wrist and down my arm. I can almost taste it. This time it's not about the kick I get out of seeing Stella's face as she catches me, just in time, dying on the floor with a

DRIPFEED

knife in my arm. This is about real pain. This physical pain redirects the pain from my heart. It makes all of it real.

Radiohead - suicide music to kill yourself to - plays in the background underneath my suicide. *Karma Police* seems fitting of the occasion. I really have given all I can, and yet it isn't enough.

After the recovery period, the weeks in hospital where Doctor Nice makes jokes about my reasons for being here, I go home. Where Stella spends her days watching me, scared that I'll do it again. Pull another stunt like that and you're dead missy. What else is left to do? Who knows? I call Ezra.

Chapter 17

Funny how karma works, isn't it? One minute you're screaming, 'I love you's' from the top of the world, and the next you're watching as your life goes down the u-bend. We had fun, as always. Whatever the weather. Whether you're lying in a ditch somewhere, smiling under some punctuating expletive, or trapped in a toilet where someone's written *blood controls everything* on a Tampax machine.

We were the people of the night; we mowed your lawns so you wouldn't have to. We walked your dogs while you were asleep. You never saw us because the night doesn't last so long. We were gone by the time the sun came up.

Ezra and I walk across Waterloo bridge, like we always do. Stand for a moment with our backs to the water, staring at the Hayward gallery, telling each other that we'll go there one day. As we always do. These empty, meaningless promises are things we do, even when we know it's bullshit.

"It's bullshit!" Ezra says. He's slurring his words now, now that he's so stoned out of his head, and I bet he can't even see the gallery, even though he's standing right in front of it. "I bet there's no one that I know now that I'll know in ten years." I don't even bother telling him that he's being totally random.

"Remember that man who died last year? The one who fell in the River Thames and you couldn't stop laughing." Ezra doesn't say anything, on account of the fact that my question wasn't really worth the effort. We are bound to each other right now, right here on this bridge with the wind and all that sentimental shit. It's almost poetic.

There is a couple at our bus stop, hugging each other. Their love warmed me a bit and for some strange reason, I started thinking about Ezra's bed, and how I haven't lain in it for ages; how we could be there right now if we weren't freezing our arses off on this bridge.

It's bizarre that I even made it here at all.

"It's well cold." Ezra isn't really telling me that it's cold, considering I'm here too; he just likes the sound of his own voice. We wait on the bridge, still with our backs to the water and take turns sipping from my hip flask. Technically speaking, liquid should quench thirst; except whisky isn't too technical a drink and I instead feel like someone emptied Brighton beach down my throat. We should have brought scarves but we never come prepared. "What's the plan Stan?" Ezra asks me.

"There isn't one. Go to yours and go to sleep. Being broke sucks, especially when I am lacking in the fundage to even leave my house."

"But you're here."

"Barely. And besides, I am completely broke now."

"Get a job," says Ezra.

"Getting a job," I say, "is way too easy."

Lami Okrekson

Ezra lights another cigarette and blows smoke rings in my face, smoke rings I breathe in and then back out again through my nose.

We walk down the steps under the bridge, near where the skater boys who don't like to be called 'skater boys' smoke spicy cigarettes and fall over. On a part that's dry, with no wind, we sit and watch them for a while. The air down here, under the road, is muggy with the aroma of boy sweat. Ezra pulls out a baggie of coke.

"Thought you quit," I say.

"Yeah," says Ezra. He doesn't bother emptying the bag into pretty white lines; the wind could come at any minute, or the skater boys. Instead he snorts the coke straight from the bag with a rolled up five pound note - adding to the ninety-nine percent of bank notes in the UK with traces of cocaine on them. The internal monologue inside my head goes into hyper drive. Is this what we've become? I mean really become. Two stoned kids doing coke under a bridge. How original.

Two of the 'skater boys' start fighting, though we don't know what it's about, and they're too far away for us to hear them properly.

"England is so fucked up," says Ezra. "I'm moving to the States."

"You think it's any less fucked up over there?" I ask. And I mean it. It really annoys me how people still buy into that American Dream bullshit when they have the highest murder rate in any other developed country. And the sickest thing in all that is that nowhere is really safe. We are destroying the world, and then we have the audacity to complain about it. We could run away to the moon but that wouldn't help. It's not the Earth, it's us.

"Oi! Fag. Give us a bit." One of the skater boys is pointing and gesturing towards the bag on the end of Ezra's nose. Ezra won't even bother telling him to fuck off. These people are not even worthy of an answer. "Come on," continues the skater boy. "I'll let you bum me."
Ezra passes the bag to me. I also promised I would quit, after the overdose. A promise can never be guaranteed, there's always an exception. And if there's any greater exception than temptation, this is it.
The skater boy continues badgering Ezra from way over by the water, but we block him out. We're good at that, blocking things out. Aside from our partying and regular drug use - insert fun illegal pastime here - the only thing we are good at is being teenagers. Isn't that what we are supposed to do anyway? If we didn't, there would be no one for the parental units to blame their heart attacks and low bank balances on. We are what is wrong with modern society. Perhaps they should bring back the cane and beat the shit out of all the unruly four year olds. Probably that will save them from a fate worse than death; it will save them from becoming us. Us vampires, people of the night and all that. The children are

not the future, they are screwed from conception. We are the future. Me and Ezra underneath Waterloo bridge with bags of cocaine attached to our noses. We are the ones who will inherit the world, if we can just make it to the other side alive.

I think the skater boy gives up asking for coke, he's too young anyway. Either way, I can't hear him anymore; though I can't hear much of anything anymore. I can't hear the wheels on the concrete, or the water. We were stoned before, now we are incredibly fucked up.

  This feels like the end of my life - like there is a full stop hanging over my head or something. I can't see where I can go from here, and I think that maybe I *am* depressed. Although *depressed* is far too strong a word to use for this. Depressed is how I felt after the summer holidays. Coming back, out of touch with everything and realising I hadn't spent enough time with the androids.

  I came back and something had changed. Some major thing, so major that I didn't even realise what was happening until I took a step back and reviewed the situation from a different perspective. You can do that, if you know how; step sideways into someone else's perspective. I looked at everything, and I looked at me, and I realised something was wrong - but I didn't know what. No one else noticed it, not Chris or Belle, not even Ezra. They all walked around like the androids I hate, smiling and carrying on as normal. I didn't know what I was feeling, and that depressed me. So I tried, for a while, to laugh at

DRIPFEED

their jokes, smoke their weed and snort their cocaine. Smiled with my mouth. But it didn't change.

Sometimes I wished they would all disappear, off to some place far, far away from me. They tired me with their energy, draining all of mine. Everything got me down. I was too young to be cynical, but already life was getting me down. I tried deluding myself, and them, which only made it worse. It was like the summer changed me somehow. Like I had been away for so long that I had forgotten how to be.

If this is the end of my life then I'm glad. I hate London. Everyone is always talking about how great London is, how privileged we are to live in Britain's capital city. Bullshit. The fact is, London sucks. And stupid people keep coming here on holiday so they can buy big union jack flags and breathe the same air they'd be breathing anywhere else.

All this time travel just wastes time.

The depression is why I'm here, why I'm this, why I'm shovelling cocaine into my nostrils when I promised them I wouldn't.

Ezra and I get up from wherever we are sitting, Ezra putting what's left of the bag in the pocket of his trench coat. We make our way back up the stairs and along the bridge. The air got colder while we were gone and the couple have disappeared. While we are waiting at the bus stop watching our breath turn to frost in air that is way too cold for September, Ezra walks into the road and gets hit by a lorry - which stops a few yards down the road.

If I was expecting anything tonight, it was not this. In fact, the only thing I'm thinking as the lorry driver runs over to check Ezra's mangled body is, "I hope they don't find the cocaine in his pocket." They'll blame me of course; they always blame someone else's child, as if their own child is too well trained to do anything worse than a hiccup in church.
    I could slip away from this scene, back under the bridge, into a club, the water - though sharks don't sleep so they'd mangle me too. I could slip, unnoticed, back into my real life, and leave Ezra and this life behind. I could but I don't. I stay and watch as the lorry driver, and then paramedics, pronounce him dead. I stay as his parents arrive, shouting things at me - things I can't hear because I am blocking them out - shoving the cocaine in my face, blaming me as I knew they would. I even stay as Stella arrives, hugging me, relived that it wasn't her kid, then shouting at me pointlessly. I stay there even when I'm not. When I'm going far away from the place I hate so much; as if that's going to make a difference. It's not the place, it's me.

I don't think about Ezra, he's fine. Life is just an old friend we visit on the way home - we never stay there long enough.

DRIPFEED

They told us the world was safe, but look at us now - friendless and running - we're dying before we've even got out of bed in the morning. We were supposed to inherit everything. They promised us the world but they fucked that up too.

www.ingramcontent.com/pod-product-compliance
Ingram Content Group UK Ltd.
Pitfield, Milton Keynes, MK11 3LW, UK
UKHW041410180426
11947UKWH00007B/46